Institute on Science for Global Policy (ISGP)

Emerging and Persistent Infectious Diseases:
Focus on Mitigation

Conference convened by the ISGP at the University of Edinburgh

Edinburgh, Scotland, United Kingdom

Oct. 23–26, 2011

An ongoing series of dialogues and critical debates
examining the role of science and technology
in advancing effective domestic and international policy decisions

Institute on Science for Global Policy (ISGP)

Tucson, AZ Office
845 N. Park Ave., 5th Floor
PO Box 210158-B
Tucson, AZ 85721

Washington, DC Office
818 Connecticut Ave. NW
Suite 800
Washington, DC 20006

www.scienceforglobalpolicy.org

ISBN: 978-0-9830882-2-6

Acknowledgment

Numerous individuals and organizations have made important contributions to the Institute on Science for Global Policy (ISGP) program on Emerging and Persistent Infectious Diseases (EPID). Some of these contributions directly supported the efforts needed to organize and convene the invitation-only ISGP conference on *EPID: Focus on Mitigation* held at the University of Edinburgh, Edinburgh, Scotland, Oct. 23–26, 2011. Other contributions aided the ISGP in preparing the material presented in this book, including not only the eight invited policy position papers, but a record, without attribution, of the views presented in the discussions, critical debates, and caucuses that ensued.

We would like to thank our colleagues at the University of Edinburgh, and especially Prof. Nigel Brown, EU Senior Vice Principal for Planning, Resources and Research Policy, for their many contributions toward the success of this conference. This conference also could not have been held without the support of our British colleagues at the Society for General Microbiology and the United Kingdom Ministry of Defence.

The process began with the early recognition that EPID and related aspects of Food Safety and Security (FSS) and Synthetic Biology (SB) are topics that deserve significantly greater attention from both domestic and international policy makers. The willingness of those in the scientific and policy communities who have expertise and experience with EPID, FSS, and SB to be interviewed by the ISGP staff was a critical early step in creating and updating the Strategic Roadmap on EPID. The resultant Strategic Roadmap describes the two-year-plus series of ISGP conferences focused on different policy aspects of EPID, FSS, and SB. The endorsement of and support for the EPID Strategic Roadmap by the governments engaged with the ISGP facilitated the launching of the EPID conference series and the convening by the ISGP of the *EPID: Focus on Mitigation* conference.

The efforts of the scientific presenters invited by the ISGP in both preparing policy position papers and engaging policy makers in vigorous debates were especially appreciated. Their biographies are provided in this book.

No less critical to the success of the program were the often-intense debates that originated among the scientific presenters and the subject-matter experts and policy makers in the audience who, following consultations with the participating governments and organizations, were invited to attend the October 2011 conference. The exchange of strongly held views, innovative proposals, and critiques generated from questions and debates fostered an unusual, even unique, environment focused on clarifying understanding for the nonspecialist and addressing specific questions related to formulating and implementing effective public policy pertaining to EPID, FSS and SB.

The ISGP is greatly indebted to all those who participated in these vigorous, not-for-attribution debates and caucuses.

The energetic, highly professional work of the ISGP staff merits special acknowledgment. Their outstanding interviewing, organizing, and writing skills were essential to recording the often-diverse views and perspectives expressed in the critical debates, capturing the areas of consensus and next steps from the caucuses, and persevering through the extensive editing process needed to assure the accuracy of the material published here. All of their work is gratefully acknowledged. Their biographies are provided in the book.

Finally, the ISGP expresses sincere appreciation for the advice and financial support of agencies and departments of the U.S. federal government including the National Intelligence Council, the Department of State, the Department of Homeland Security, and the Department of Health and Human Services — Assistant Secretary for Preparedness and Response. Major scientific and financial support was also provided by the Istituto Regionale di Ricerca in Milan, Italy. The ISGP also benefited from the recommendations and generous gifts provided by the MARS Corp., Novartis, GlaxoSmithKline, and Mr. Edward Bessey. The ISGP gratefully acknowledges the ongoing support provided by the Critical Path Institute, the University of Arizona, and the University of Minnesota.

Dr. George H. Atkinson
Founder and Executive Director
Institute on Science for Global Policy
February 13, 2012

Table of contents

Introduction
Dr. George H. Atkinson
Founder and Executive Director, Institute on Science for Global Policy
and
Professor, Department of Chemistry and Biochemistry,
College of Optical Sciences,
and College of Science, University of Arizona

Preface

The contents of this book were taken from material presented at an international conference convened by the Institute on Science for Global Policy (ISGP) on Oct. 23–26, 2011, in Scotland at the University of Edinburgh. This ISGP conference specifically addressed topics involving the mitigation of Emerging and Persistent Infectious Diseases (EPID) as well as aspects of Food Safety and Security (FSS) and Synthetic Biology (SB) related to infectious diseases. The material in this book includes policy position papers prepared by eight internationally distinguished subject-matter experts in these fields together with the not-for-attribution summaries prepared by the ISGP staff of the discussions, debates, and caucuses that comprised important parts of the ISGP conference. While the material presented here is comprehensive and stands by itself, its policy significance is best appreciated if viewed within the context of how domestic and international science policies have been, and often currently are being, formulated and implemented.

Current realities

As the second decade of the 21st century opens, most societies are facing difficult decisions concerning how to appropriately use, or reject, the dramatic new opportunities offered by modern scientific advances and the technologies that emanate from them. Advanced scientific research programs, as well as commercially viable technologies, are now developed globally. As a consequence, many societal issues related to science and technology (S&T) necessarily involve both domestic and international policy decisions. The daunting challenges to simultaneously recognize immediate technological opportunities, while identifying those emerging and "at-the-horizon" S&T achievements that foreshadow transformational advantages and risks within specific societies, are now fundamental governmental responsibilities. These responsibilities are especially complex since policy makers must consider the demands of different segments of society, which often have conflicting goals. For example, decisions must balance critical commercial interests that promote economic prosperity with the cultural sensitivities that often determine if, and how, S&T can be successfully integrated into any society.

Many of our most significant geopolitical policy and security issues are directly connected with the remarkably rapid and profound S&T accomplishments of our time. Consequently, it is increasingly important that the S&T and policy communities communicate effectively. With a seemingly unlimited number of urgent S&T challenges, both wealthy and less-wealthy societies need the most accomplished members of these communities to focus on effective, real-world solutions relevant to their specific circumstances. Some of the most prominent challenges involve (i) infectious diseases and pandemics, (ii) environmentally compatible energy sources, (iii) the consequences of climate change, (iv) food safety and security, (v) the cultural impact of stem cell applications, (vi) nanotechnology and human health, (vii) cyber security for advanced telecommunication, (viii) the security implications of quantum computing, and (ix) the cultural radicalization of societies.

Recent history suggests that most societies would benefit from improving the effectiveness of how scientifically credible information is used to formulate and implement governmental policies, both domestic and international. Specifically, there is a critical need to have the relevant S&T information concisely presented to policy communities in an environment that promotes candid questions and debates led by those non-experts directly engaged in decisions. Such discussions, sequestered away from publicity, can help to clarify the advantages and potential risks of realistic S&T options directly relevant to the challenges being faced. Eventually, this same degree of understanding, confidence, and acknowledgment of risk must be communicated to the public to obtain the broad societal support needed to effectively implement any decision.

The ISGP mission

The Institute on Science for Global Policy (ISGP) has pioneered the development of a new type of international forum based on a series of invitation-only conferences. These ISGP conferences are designed to provide articulate, distinguished scientists and technologists opportunities to concisely present their views of the credible S&T options available for addressing major geopolitical and security issues. Over a two-year period, these ISGP conferences are convened on different aspects (e.g., surveillance, prevention, or mitigation) of a broad, overarching topic (currently, EPID and related aspects of FSS and SB). The format used emphasizes written and oral, policy-oriented S&T presentations and extensive debates led by an international cross section of the policy community.

The current realities, relevant S&T-based options (including risks), and policy issues are debated among a few scientists selected by the ISGP and an international group of government, private sector, and societal leaders selected following consultations with the participating governments and organizations. ISGP conferences reflect global perspectives and seek to provide government and community leaders with the clear, accurate understanding of the real-world challenges and potential solutions critical to determining sound public policies.

ISGP programs rely on the validity of two overarching principles:

1.   Scientifically credible understanding must be closely linked to the realistic policy decisions made by governmental and societal leaders in addressing both the urgent and long-term challenges facing 21st century societies. Effective decisions rely on strong domestic and global public endorsements that motivate active support throughout societies.

2.   Communication among scientific and policy communities requires significant improvement, especially concerning decisions on whether to use or reject the often transformational scientific and technological opportunities continually emerging from the global research communities. Effective decisions are facilitated in venues where the advantages and risks of credible options are candidly presented and critically debated among internationally distinguished subject-matter experts, policy makers, and private sector and community stakeholders.

Historical perspective

The dramatic and rapid expansion of academic and private sector scientific research transformed many societies of the 20th century and is a major factor in the emergence of the more affluent countries that currently dominate the global economic and security landscape. The positive influence of these S&T achievements has been extremely impressive and in many ways the hallmark of the 20th century. However, there have also been numerous negative consequences, some immediately apparent and others appearing only recently. From both perspectives, it would be difficult to argue that S&T has not been the prime factor defining the societies we know today. Indeed, the 20th century can be viewed through the prism of how societies decided to use the available scientific understanding and technological expertise to structure themselves. Such decisions helped shape the respective economic models, cultural priorities, and security commitments in these societies.

It remains to be seen how the prosperity and security of 21st century societies will be shaped by the decisions made by our current leaders, especially with respect to how these decisions reflect sound S&T understanding.

Given the critical importance of properly incorporating scientifically credible information into major societal decisions, it is surprising that the process by which this is achieved by the public and its political leadership has been uneven and, occasionally, haphazard. In the worst cases, decisions have been based on unrecognized misunderstanding, overhyped optimism, and/or limited respect for potentially negative consequences. Retrospectively, while some of these outcomes may be attributed to politically motivated priorities, the inability of S&T experts to accurately communicate the advantages and potential risks of a given option must also be acknowledged as equally important.

The new format pioneered by the ISGP in its programs seeks to facilitate candid communication between scientific and policy communities in ways that complement and support the efforts of others.

It is important to recognize that policy makers routinely seek a degree of certainty in evaluating S&T-based options that is inconsistent with reality, while S&T experts often overvalue the potentially positive aspects of their proposals. Finite uncertainty is always part of advanced scientific thinking and all possible positive outcomes in S&T proposals are rarely realized. Both points need to be reflected in policy decisions. Eventually, the public needs to be given a frank, accurate assessment of the potential advantages and foreseeable disadvantages associated with these decisions. Such disclosures are essential to obtain the broad public support required to effectively implement any major decision.

ISGP conference structure

At each ISGP conference, eight internationally recognized, subject-matter experts are invited to prepare concise (three pages) policy position papers. For the Oct. 23–26, 2011, ISGP conference in Scotland, these papers described the authors' views on current realities, scientifically credible opportunities and associated risks, and policy issues involved in the mitigation of EPID, the promotion of FSS and the productive development of SB.

These eight authors were chosen to represent a broad cross section of viewpoints and an international perspective. Several weeks before the conference convened, these policy position papers were distributed to representatives from governments, societal organizations, and international organizations engaged with the ISGP (the United States, Italy, the United Kingdom, Japan, Canada, France, Mexico, Germany, the Food and Agricultural Organization of the United Nations, and the European Commission). Individuals from several private sector and philanthropic organizations also were invited to participate and, therefore, received the papers. All participants had responsibilities and/or made major contributions to the formulation and implementation of domestic and international policies related to EPID, FSS, and SB.

The conference agenda was comprised of eight 90-minute sessions, each of which was devoted to a debate of a given policy position paper. To encourage frank discussions and critical debates, all ISGP conferences are conducted under the Chatham House Rule (i.e., all the information can be used freely, but there can be no attribution of any remark to any participant). In each session, the author was given 5 minutes to summarize his or her views while the remaining 85 minutes were opened to all participants, including other authors, for questions, comments, and debate. The focus was on obtaining clarity of understanding among the nonspecialists and identifying areas of consensus and actionable policy decisions supported by scientifically credible information. With active participation from North America, Europe, and Asia, these candid debates are designed to reflect international perspectives on real-world problems.

The ISGP staff attended the debates of all eight policy position papers. The "not-for-attribution" summaries of each debate, prepared from their collective notes, are presented here immediately following each policy position paper. These summaries represent the ISGP's best effort to accurately capture the comments and questions made by the participants, including the other authors, as well as those responses made by the author of the paper. The views expressed in these summaries do not necessarily represent the views of a specific author, as evidenced by his or her respective policy position paper. Rather, the summaries are, and should be read as, an overview of the areas of agreement and disagreement that emerged from all those participating in the debates.

Following the eight debates, caucuses were held by small groups each representing a cross section of the participants. A separate caucus for the scientific presenters also was held. These caucuses focused on identifying areas of consensus and actionable next steps for consideration within governments and civil societies in general. Subsequently, a plenary caucus was convened for all participants. While the debates focused on specific issues and recommendations raised in each policy position paper, the caucuses focused on overarching views and conclusions that could have policy relevance both domestically and internationally.

A summary of the overall areas of consensus and actionable next steps emerging from these caucuses is presented here immediately following this introduction under the title of **Conference conclusions.**

Concluding remarks

ISGP conferences are designed to provide new and unusual (perhaps unique) environments that facilitate and encourage candid debate of the credible S&T options vital to successfully address many of the most significant challenges facing 21st century societies. ISGP debates test the views of subject-matter experts through critical questions and comments from an international group of decision makers committed to finding effective, real-world solutions. Obviously, ISGP conferences build on the authoritative reports and expertise expressed by many domestic and international organizations already actively devoted to this task. The ISGP has no preconceived opinions nor do members of the ISGP staff express any independent views on these topics. Rather, ISGP programs focus on fostering environments that can significantly improve the communication of ideas and recommendations, many of which are in reports developed by other organizations and institutes, to the policy communities responsible for serving their constituents.

ISGP conferences begin with concise descriptions of scientifically credible options provided by those experienced in the S&T subject, but rely heavily on the willingness of nonspecialists in government, academe, foundations, and the private sector to critically debate these S&T concepts and proposals. Overall, ISGP conferences seek to provide a new type of venue in which S&T expertise not only informs the nonspecialists, but also in which the debates and caucuses identify realistic policy options for serious consideration by governments and societal leaders. These new ISGP programs can help ensure that S&T understanding is integrated into those real-world policy decisions needed to foster safer and more prosperous 21st century societies.

Conference conclusions

Area of consensus 1:

Since infectious diseases do not respect borders, it is critical for all mitigation efforts that the relevant data, knowledge, and materials be shared throughout intergovernmental agencies, among societal organizations, and across international borders in a timely and transparent manner. For such efforts to be successful, it is essential that data standards reflect diverse international perspectives and that sufficient financial resources be committed through anticipatory, proactive policies.

Actionable next steps:

1. The effectiveness of communication of prioritized baseline data (e.g., human case rates and demographic characteristics, animal case rates and geographic locations, emerging symptoms) among all infectious disease surveillance systems must be strengthened in a manner that is consistent with One Health models. The creation and implementation of a common global database system would improve the management and sharing of such surveillance data for mitigation. Flexible standards that better harmonize surveillance data, while integrating information from new technologies, are key elements in constructing useful databases.

2. The ongoing debates over intellectual property rights, biopiracy, and ownership of data and materials related to infectious diseases emphasizes the need to balance the benefits accruing to the global scientific community with those accruing to local, regional and national groups.

Area of consensus 2:

It is generally recognized that the compartmentalization of surveillance data, analysis information, and mitigation efforts within segmented governmental and societal groups (i.e., siloization) routinely causes mitigation efforts for infectious diseases to be disjointed and duplicative. Strengthening the coordination across professional disciplines (e.g., animal and human health), across agencies and programs within agencies, among countries, and especially between private and public entities is a critical aspect for improving the effectiveness of mitigation policies. Even coordination within a discipline (e.g., virology) is often absent.

Actionable next steps:

1. Infectious disease control should be approached in the context of One Health concepts in which disease-specific approaches using this multidisciplinary framework (e.g., "One Flu") are used. Infectious disease mitigation strategies can only be effective if such an integrated, multidisciplinary structure is adopted.

2. Although individual disciplinary groups (e.g., virology) have often responded well to outbreaks of new infectious diseases (e.g., Severe Acute Respiratory Syndrome [SARS]), a successful response cannot be guaranteed without enhanced, proactive coordination within professional disciplines. Improved, proactive coordination of responses within disciplinary laboratories and strong interdisciplinary training of young scientists are necessary to ensure a rapid and successful response to disease outbreaks.

Area of consensus 3:

The globalization of the world's food supply and the associated homogenization of food sources have significantly reduced costs and expanded access, but have also increased exposure to foodborne diseases. In an increasingly globalized food supply chain driven by consumer demands, there exists a greater emphasis on the need for food safety regulations that reflect cultural differences and which are supported through both public policies and private sector practices.

Actionable next steps:

1. The worldwide harmonization of food safety standards is critical for a food supply chain that is increasingly globalized. It is equally critical that producers are able to finance the increased costs associated with improved food safety standards if a competitive global market is to be maintained.

2. Improvements in food testing methods needed to facilitate early pathogen detection, including advanced real-time diagnostics and sampling, can have a profound impact on food safety. The new information available from these advanced capabilities requires policy makers and food industry stakeholders to better understand the food supply as it relates to the traceability of products and ingredients to their points of manufacture and sources. Public-private cooperation

on food safety, including the transparent and timely sharing of data, must be significantly strengthened if both the public safety and private sector economic interests are to be protected by accurately and rapidly characterizing the increasing appearances of serious foodborne diseases.

3. While consumers do not consistently recognize and/or accept the risks associated with their consumption of certain food products, public health officials, regulatory agencies, and the private sector are increasingly responsible for providing accurate and timely food safety information that relates to infectious disease outbreaks. Such messages must be tailored to effectively communicate with individuals across different cultures, socioeconomic backgrounds, and geographies.

4. Incorrect and excessive use of antibiotics in food production require that veterinarians have comprehensive oversight on how and when antibiotics are used and that food producers are educated concerning the importance of correct antibiotic practices, including the proper restriction of imported products known to be problematic.

Area of consensus 4:

Applications of synthetic biology offer the potential for profound advances in the mitigation of infectious diseases through the design, redesign, and fabrication of biological parts, devices, and systems (e.g., vaccines, pharmaceuticals, diagnostics, re-engineered vectors). As part of the newest examples of genetic engineering, technologies based on synthetic biology can accelerate, reduce the cost, and broaden the scale of such developments. As with all advanced technologies, the safe and ethical use of these opportunities, including both accidental or intentional misuse, requires proactive discussions among the global synthetic biology communities and their respective governmental and societal representatives to balance safety with innovation.

Actionable next steps:

1. Effective approaches to addressing safety and ethical concerns related to synthetic biology activities require that the need to protect the public from potential misuse is balanced with regulatory policies and practices that do not constrain the scientific advancements needed to control diseases and to respond against intentionally harmful applications of synthetic biology. Scientists in the private sector, academia, and government laboratories must develop ethical codes of conduct and

practical indicators (e.g., screening oligonucleotide purchases) that minimize the potential risks associated with the nefarious uses of synthetic biology.

2.   To ensure that its impact on disease mitigation is fully realized, the public perceptions of risk must be consistent with the realities of risk associated with synthetic biology activities. To avoid the negative consequences of past experiences (e.g., genetically modified organisms or GMOs), the true nature of potential hazards must be accurately and promptly understood by policy makers and candidly conveyed to the public.

Area of consensus 5:

Characteristics of the 21st century information and technology environment have complicated efforts to accurately and effectively communicate risk, which has caused the public to face difficulties distinguishing fact from opinion, inaccurately perceive risk, and experience confusion about which health recommendations to follow. Risk communication to both the public and policy makers must be based on scientific research such that a determination of effective messages and appropriate communication formats and platforms can be made.

Actionable next steps:

1.   Science-based communication of risk related to mitigating diseases, both prior to and during a crisis, must be credibly conveyed by trusted sources and must be tailored to address the public's diverse values, beliefs, concerns, perceptions of risk, customs, and agendas. As such, risk communication needs to consider: i) the content of the message and how it is framed, ii) how the content is presented, through numbers, facts, and/or stories, and iii) the dissemination channels used such as mobile phones, Internet, and/or television/film.

2.   Relationships among trusted scientific, public, and media leaders need to be established well in advance of a disease emergency to ensure that scientifically credible evidence is consistently and transparently presented to the public. Specific attention needs to be devoted to: i) explaining the models used to help mitigate infectious disease outbreaks and their limitations, ii) minimizing ambiguity in the advice presented to the

public (e.g., avoid simultaneously advising the public to conduct "business as usual" and to stay away from work), and iii) using social networking technologies for disseminating information.

3. Given that effective risk communication must be a core competency for all involved in protecting public health, media and risk communication training of science and medical graduates, public health professionals, policy makers, and all prospective crisis spokespeople needs to be given a high priority.

ISGP conference program

Sunday, Oct. 23

12:00 – 17:00   **Arrival and Registration: John McIntyre Conference Centre, Pollock Halls, University of Edinburgh**

16:30 – 17:30   **Caucus Meeting**

17:30 – 19:00   *Reception*

19:00 – 20:00   *Dinner*

20:00 – 20:45   **Welcome and Opening Remarks**
Dr. George Atkinson, Founder and Executive Director, ISGP, and Conference Moderator

Monday, Oct. 24

08:00 – 08:45   *Breakfast*

Presentations and Debates: Session 1

09:00 – 10:30   **Dr. Ilaria Capua, Istituto Zooprofilattico Sperimentale delle Venezie, Italy**
It's Not What You Know, But What You Do With What You Know

10:30 – 11:00   *Break*

11:00 – 12:30   **Prof. Robert Gallo, University of Maryland School of Medicine and Global Virus Network, United States**
The Need for Expanded Global Efforts to Mitigate Viral Threats: Lessons from the HIV/AIDS Epidemic

12:30 – 13:30   *Lunch*

13:30 – 14:00   **Informal Discussion: 2012 ISGP Programs**

Presentations and Debates: Session 2

14:00 – 15:30   **Prof. Kasisomayajula "Vish" Viswanath, Harvard School of Public Health, Dana-Farber Cancer Institute, and Dana-Farber/Harvard Cancer Center, United States**
Communicating Risk in the Age of Information Plenty: Implication for Policy and Practice of Emerging and Persistent Infectious Diseases (EPID)

15:30 – 16:00   *Break*

16:00 – 17:30   **Prof. Sir Roy Anderson, Imperial College London, United Kingdom**
Planning for Pandemics: The Formulation of Policy

19:00 – 21:00   *Dinner, Playfair Library, Edinburgh*

Tuesday, Oct. 25

08:00 – 08:45   *Breakfast*

Presentations and Debates: Session 3

09:00 – 10:30   **Prof. Shaun Kennedy, National Center for Food Protection and Defense and University of Minnesota, United States**
Proactive Use of Supply Chain Data in Foodborne Illness Outbreak Investigation

10:30 – 11:00   *Break*

11:00 – 12:30   **Dr. Michael Doyle, University of Georgia, United States**
Opportunities for Mitigating Foodborne Illnesses Caused by Emerging and Persistent Infectious Agents

12:30 – 13:30   *Lunch*

13:30 – 14:00   **Informal Discussion: 2012 ISGP Programs**

Presentations and Debates: Session 4

14:00 – 15:30   **Dr. John Glass, J. Craig Venter Institute, United States**
Synthetic Biology: A New Weapon in Our War Against Infectious Diseases

15:30 – 16:00   *Break*

16:00 – 17:30   **Prof. Joyce Tait, University of Edinburgh, United Kingdom**
Innovation, Policy, and Public Interactions in the Management of Infectious Diseases

Caucuses

17:00 – 21:30   **Focused group sessions**

Wednesday, Oct. 26

08:00 – 08:45   *Breakfast*

09:00 – 10:45   **Plenary session**
Dr. George Atkinson, *moderator*

10:45 – 11:00   *Break*

11:00 – 12:30   **Policy Panel: Comments and questions**
Dr. George Atkinson, *moderator*

12:30 – 12:40   **Closing Remarks**
Dr. George Atkinson

12:40-13:30   *Lunch*

13:30   *Adjournment*

It's Not What You Know, But What You Do With What You Know[**]

Ilaria Capua, D.V.M., Ph.D.
Director, Division of Comparative Biomedical Sciences,
Istituto Zooprofilattico Sperimentale delle Venezie, Padova, Italy

Summary

Two and a half years after the emergence of the first pandemic influenza virus of the 21st century, we are certain there is space for improvement in the area of preparedness, and thus for mitigation. The persistence of a dogmatic approach for controlling factors underlying the emergence of influenza virus strains that are capable of both jumping the species barrier and spreading among human populations has produced negative outcomes. Such consequences range from mistrust of public health authorities to the delayed availability of vaccines. For this reason, our prediction skills must be improved, and the first step in this direction is to be able to comprehensively analyze the pandemic potential of animal influenza viruses. Paradoxically, we have the dataset, but we just do not look at it with the appropriate tools and mindset. What we need is a "One Flu" approach. This approach includes the development of a permanent observatory (either virtual or physical), including analytic tools that can identify and grade animal strains that fulfill some or all the requisites of a pandemic virus before the virus becomes a problem in humans. This would enable us to have a library of "potentially pandemic" strains which can be used as seeds for vaccine manufacture to ensure product availability in a shorter period of time. The creation of an interdisciplinary data library requires an ongoing and timely mechanism to ensure transparency between the veterinary and medical communities on genetic and epidemiological data, which are routinely collected through surveillance efforts worldwide; such a library is in line with the "One Health" vision. This interdisciplinary approach would pave the way for similar methodologies applicable to other emerging and zoonotic infectious diseases, thus complementing other efforts in the fields of preparedness, response, and mitigation.

Current realities

More than two years after the emergence and spread of the first influenza pandemic of the new millennium, we are aware of how our prediction skills need to improve on many fronts. The emergence of the H1N1 virus strain responsible for the 2009 influenza pandemic (PDM 2009 H1N1) was an unexpected event for most influenza scientists. The viral subtype and the geographical and biological origin of the virus were distant from both the geographic regions and the areas of research where significant funds for influenza were invested. The influenza epicenter was deemed to be Southeast Asia, and the epizootic of a highly virulent H5N1, with a previously unseen capacity to jump the species barrier, was believed to be the most likely candidate for the next human pandemic.

In reality, PDM 2009 H1N1 originated from Central America rather than Southeast Asia. Additionally, PDM 2009 H1N1 was of a subtype not included in the pre-pandemic candidate list, was relatively mild (compared to the virulence of H5N1), and emerged from swine rather than birds. In hindsight, the pandemic potential of some animal viruses was underestimated. These examples illustrate the importance of improving our prediction skills.

Until 2009, the real and perceived threat posed by H5N1 viruses had drawn significant resources to issues related to avian influenza viruses, particularly in Eurasia. Influenza infections in mammalian species were neglected, particularly in the Americas. In addition, a rather dogmatic approach suggested that to ignite a pandemic, the virus had to be of a different subtype than those that were circulating in the human population as seasonal strains. These two blind spots impeded the identification of the emerging risk in Central America.

Possibly the only correct prediction attempt was that a new pandemic virus would very rapidly infect the entire world population, exploiting opportunities offered by globalization. Although PDM 2009 H1N1 is considered a relatively mild pandemic, it resulted in significant mortality data and years of life lost. Had there been a suitable pre-pandemic vaccine available in time, morbidity and mortality could have been greatly reduced.

In addition, "betting on the wrong virus" (i.e., H5N1) has caused a general sense of mistrust of international health organizations and resulted in avoidable damages to the perception of international health policies aimed at preparedness and mitigation.

Scientific opportunities and challenges

Looking to the future, it is important to bear in mind that we may be baffled again by this disease. Although the recent pandemic was not as severe as had been envisaged for a pandemic caused by H5N1, the future occurrence of a severe influenza pandemic cannot be ruled out. Avian viruses (e.g., H5N1) and others with zoonotic potential (e.g., H9N2) are still endemic in large portions of the eastern hemisphere. Swine influenza viruses and other mammalian viruses are also circulating at a global level, and together with viruses of wild and domestic poultry, represent a unique evolving gene pool containing the precursors of the next human pandemic strain.

We have to recognize that vast improvements in capacity building have been achieved as a result of the H5N1 global crisis. Investments in infrastructure and training have yielded a network of scientists with improved influenza diagnostic capacity. Thousands of viral isolates with zoonotic potential have been obtained through surveillance efforts. However, the genetic information has not been fully exploited. An in-depth knowledge of these viruses would allow the scientific community to obtain a better picture of the pandemic potential of selected strains, and enable the development of better prevention and mitigation strategies.

Influenza infections still represent a major threat to mankind, to the livelihood of rural villages, and to the health and productivity of animals. The recent pandemic highlights a need to improve our prediction capacities to enact more efficient prevention strategies through integrated research and surveillance efforts, embracing both animal health and public health. This is in line with, and possibly the best example of, the One Health vision: a multidisciplinary collaborative approach to improve the health of humans, animals, and the environment, endorsed by the Food & Agriculture Organization of the United Nations (FAO), the World Organisation for Animal Health (OIE), and the World Health Organization (WHO). The One Flu initiative would result in international synergies, bridging gaps between medical and veterinary scientists, permanent monitoring of virus evolution and epidemiology, and the best exploitation of investments in capacity building. Above all, it would be a challenge and an opportunity to apply a One Health approach to influenza (i.e., One Flu). Moreover, this approach could possibly act as a model for other emerging zoonotic diseases.

Policy issues

- A permanent observatory that contains existing genetic and epidemiological information on strains that are collected globally through animal and human surveillance efforts must be developed. Such an observatory would provide a basis for a more educated approach to assessing the pandemic potential of currently circulating viruses. Furthermore, it would enable the identification of potential pandemic precursors as they exist in nature. Identifying the pandemic potential of viruses can be achieved by analyzing the wealth of existing genetic and epidemiologic information to determine which risk factors are likely responsible for the transmission and severity of disease in humans.

- International organizations such as FAO, OIE, and WHO should fortify their surveillance efforts through existing mechanisms, particularly in neglected geographical areas and animal species.
- International donors and funding agencies involved in influenza research and surveillance efforts should ensure that data generated through their funding is made readily available to the scientific community in an equitable, ethical, and efficient manner, as recommended by Walport and Brest (2011).
- Full genome sequencing of influenza viruses should be performed on isolates collected through routine and targeted surveillance, and these sequences should be compulsorily made available in the public domain in a timely manner.
- Entities that hold genetic and epidemiological databases for influenza viruses should ensure compatibility with other datasets and invest in software that can screen sequences for relevant mutations.
- An international One Flu effort should be pursued by relevant public health organizations. This effort should include the use of a flexible risk assessment framework, capable of identifying and grading the pandemic risk posed by selected animal influenza viruses.

References

World Health Organization. (2011, April 17). *Landmark agreement improves global preparedness for influenza pandemics.* [News release]. Retrieved September 9, 2011, from http://www.who.int/mediacentre/news/releases/2011/pandemic_influenza_prep_ 20110417/en/index.html

Walport, M. & Brest, P. (2011). Sharing research data to improve public health. *The Lancet, 377*(9765), 537–39.

Istituto Zooprofilattico Sperimentale delle Venezie in collaboration with CDC's Influenza Division/NCIRD and the One Health Office. (2011). *Executive summary of the One Flu Strategic Retreat, February 1–3, 2011, Treviso, Italy.* Retrieved August 9, 2011, from http://www.cdc.gov/onehealth/pdf/castelbrando/executive-summary.pdf

*** A policy position paper prepared for presentation at the conference on Emerging and Persistent Infectious Diseases (EPID): Focus on Mitigation convened by the Institute on Science for Global Policy (ISGP) Oct. 23–26, 2011, at the University of Edinburgh, Edinburgh, Scotland.*

Debate Summary

The following summary is based on notes recorded by the ISGP staff during the not-for-attribution debate of the policy position paper prepared by Dr. Ilaria Capua (see above). Dr. Capua initiated the debate with a 5-minute statement of her views and then actively engaged the conference participants, including other authors, throughout the remainder of the 90-minute period. This Debate Summary represents the ISGP's best effort to accurately capture the comments offered and questions posed by all participants, as well as those responses made by Dr. Capua. Given the not-for-attribution format of the debate, the views comprising this summary do not necessarily represent the views of Dr. Capua, as evidenced by her policy position paper. Rather, it is, and should be read as, an overview of the areas of agreement and disagreement that emerged from all those participating in the critical debate.

Debate conclusions

- The "One Flu" approach for influenza may represent a good model for implementing a "One Health" paradigm that encompasses wildlife, domestic animal, and human health. The appropriate role for international organizations and donor bodies in this framework needs to be determined.
- Numerous barriers exist in the development and production processes intended to rapidly provide vaccines for the public, including scientific and technical limitations, strategic and political considerations, infrastructure requirements, and regulatory bottlenecks.
- While the sharing of sequence data is important, the ability to use this information to predict zoonotic potential or pathogenicity remains a key scientific challenge.
- Efforts to increase the sharing of data on animal and human diseases must consider intellectual property constraints, including uncertainties related to the ownership of strains and sequence data, and concerns (especially in less-wealthy countries) regarding access to products developed from shared information. Intellectual property discussions need to distinguish economic considerations from those issues viewed as contributing to the "global good."

- Synthetic biology offers the potential to significantly increase the scale and speed of vaccine development and manufacturing, but it is critical that the major concerns regarding biosecurity and biodefense are thoroughly addressed.

Current realities

The discussion primarily focused on efforts to mitigate the impact of influenza viruses that can cause sporadic disease as well as pandemics. Several prominent outbreaks of the H5N1 "avian" influenza strain and the 2009 "swine" influenza pandemic (PDM 2009 H1N1) illustrated the serious impact that influenza has on human welfare. The global consequences of H5N1 included significant morbidity, the loss of lives, and negative economic ramifications. While PDM 2009 H1N1 was thought to be anticlimactic in terms of morbidity and mortality, it was considered a good example of the negative economic impact that influenza can have even when pandemics are not severe.

By contrast to PDM 2009 H1N1, the recent spread of H5N1 was considered a "game changer" because it attracted international attention from donors and organizations, leading these groups to realize the importance of ensuring that medical and veterinary communities work closely together. Yet, the global focus on H5N1 as the next pandemic overshadowed other potential hazards and caused the scientific community to overlook the threat of H1N1. Although some researchers in the veterinary community, particularly in Europe, had called for increased surveillance in pigs, such surveillance did not occur on a global scale. This mismatch between where surveillance was concentrated (Southeast Asia) and where H1N1 appeared (Mexico) demonstrated the need to significantly improve our ability to predict the emergence not only of influenza, but other infectious diseases as well.

The role of data sharing in influenza prevention and mitigation provides an historical example relevant to all disease surveillance efforts. It is clear that countries, organizations, and individual scientists have long been reluctant to share their data and analyses. Such reluctance has been driven by a variety of disincentives. For example, based on several prominent events, countries were concerned that sharing their information would be more damaging than beneficial to their infectious disease control efforts. After sharing a strain of influenza, Vietnam received no advantage for its efforts, but rather was required to purchase vaccine made from the strain it isolated and shared. Many countries, accordingly, do not share the data on diseases available to them as a contribution to "global good" and now require an agreement concerning what rights they have to obtaining the benefits from the ultimate use of that data. Likewise, many scientists have guarded their genetic sequences to protect the originality of their research for academic publishing.

Although resistance to data sharing continues, the growing need for cooperation in infectious disease control is driving increased exchanges of information. This was demonstrated by efforts of the National Institute of Allergy and Infectious Diseases (NIAID) of the National Institutes of Health (NIH) to promote depositing data in the public domain. Similarly, the World Health Organization's (WHO) pandemic influenza preparedness (PIP) framework for the sharing of influenza viruses and access to vaccines and other benefits was also considered a positive step toward increased data sharing.

As a critical aspect of data sharing, intellectual property was believed to be in need of attention, especially with respect to distinguishing what constitutes a discovery versus what is defined as an invention. It was argued that gene sequences of a virus fall under the rubric of discovery because they are products of nature and the sequences can easily be re-derived. Invention was defined as a method used to create a product based on an understanding of the gene sequences. This distinction was illustrated by the U.S. Food and Drug Administration's (FDA) protocols, which categorize vaccines as a biological component (i.e., discovery), and the process of generating the vaccine as the intellectual property component (i.e., invention). However, it was strongly held that there continue to be global disagreements on where intellectual property rights for viral sequences should be conferred. The concept of "ownership" is the main issue underlying this distinction primarily because ownership designation dictates who will secure the monetary profits from a particular enterprise.

The time required to make effective vaccines available to the public is another critical factor to be considered. As a recent example, the speed with which the vaccine for PDM 2009 H1N1 was supplied to the distributors was considered slower than what is required to adequately protect the public. If the PDM 2009 H1NI strain had been more virulent, the delay in delivering the vaccine could have seriously impacted human health. It was suggested that the vaccines were not delayed because of the time it takes to produce the seed strain, but rather, because of the length of time it takes to (i) identify the production standards, (ii) bulk the vaccine strains and (iii) pass the vaccine through the regulatory process.

There was substantial debate about the development and regulation of vaccines in response to pandemic influenza. In terms of development, existing synthetic biology technology facilitates the relatively fast and inexpensive creation of influenza vaccines by using platforms that are not egg-based. An influenza virus can now be created from a DNA sequence in less than five days by advanced synthetic biology researchers. However, technology based on synthetic biology has not been universally implemented. Regardless of whether synthetic biology techniques are utilized, regulatory approval and onerous requirements associated with ensuring quality control for vaccines (particularly for those produced in less-wealthy countries) are roadblocks to rapid vaccine production.

Scientific opportunities and challenges

Despite growing acceptance of the importance of a "One Health" approach (i.e., the integration of wildlife, animal, and human health), the practical implementation of these principles has been slow. The "One Flu" approach for influenza was viewed as a good starting model for more effectively launching One Health paradigms. While it was generally agreed that influenza provides a potentially fruitful avenue for One Health implementation because of the established understanding of influenza virology and epidemiology, some concern was expressed that unknowns related to influenza virus biology (e.g., the difficulty relating sequence to pathogenicity) suggest that a more predictable disease would provide a better starting point.

While One Flu would facilitate a more holistic animal/human approach to influenza control efforts, several additional scientific challenges were identified. One Flu programs would collect sequence data and curate strains from influenza viruses in animal populations to better understand and predict how and when the virus might jump to human populations. However, current scientific capabilities do not allow the relation of sequence data to the pathogenicity of a microbe. While the current focus is only on collecting and sharing sequence data, other information (e.g., immunogenicity data) is needed.

To improve data access, it was proposed that data funded with public resources be made available in the public domain. Making data publicly available could pose a biodefense threat (e.g., by facilitating the use of sequence data for harmful purposes). However, it was noted that parameters can be placed on access, as well as on who is considered to be within the public domain, (e.g., password-protected portals can be used that only allow individuals affiliated with certain institutions to obtain the information). Additionally, it was noted that there are numerous logistical challenges that complicate widespread dissemination of and access to public domain data, including: managing large data volumes, integrating data, developing access tools, and creating metadata. Despite such concerns and challenges, U.S. efforts to promote public domain data were cited as an example of progress in this arena (e.g., U.S. requirements attached to publicly funded data have yielded almost 9,000 sequences of influenza in the public domain) and were lauded for improving researchers' access to data that can be used to improve influenza mitigation.

Although many positive aspects of mandatory data sharing were discussed, it was also noted that the governmental shift from a voluntary system to an institutional process can lead to perceptions of intrusion. Creating a compulsory structure that does not challenge privacy rights and threaten sovereignty was considered desirable but involves ongoing challenges that need to be considered early in the formulation of processes.

Increased scientific capacity was considered necessary to effectively utilize sequence data and other information accumulated through increased sharing. Predicting the ability of an influenza strain to jump the species barrier (e.g., from birds or pigs to humans) using viral sequence data was identified as a key scientific challenge. Predictions based on sequence data concerning diseases that are transmitted from wild and domestic animals to humans is a broader challenge to be applied to other zoonotic pathogens. In addition, predicting the likelihood of pathogenicity from sequence data was seen as an important capability to develop. Additionally, there exists a need to collect and curate not only data, but also physical material in the form of viral strains.

Participants discussed several opportunities and challenges related to the use of synthetic biology. Synthetic biology can be utilized to speed the production of influenza vaccines, while at the same time optimizing the amount of vaccine that is manufactured. This increased volume was illustrated by the current construction of a new Biosafety Level-3 (BSL3) facility in the U.S. This plant will be able to produce 100 to 150 million doses of tripartite vaccine twice annually (once for the northern hemisphere and once for the southern hemisphere). Although synthetic biology offers enormous opportunities for vaccine development, widespread data sharing of genetic sequences could become problematic as synthetic biology knowledge and capabilities become both more sophisticated and easier to execute. Such concern stems from fears that individuals with malicious intent would be able to easily access the information required to genetically engineer a pathogen for harmful uses.

There was also debate regarding whether a panel of influenza seed vaccines (i.e., a library of strains) should be created that could be developed quickly once a pandemic strain was identified. While the expertise exists to create a collection of pre-pandemic candidates, it was argued that it would be preferable to continue making educated decisions regarding which strains are most likely to ignite a pandemic. Because technologies like synthetic biology have so greatly accelerated the speed within which wild-type strains can be produced in forms for vaccine manufacturing, it was suggested that the need for a library has become obsolete.

Policy issues

It was widely agreed that increased efforts to address intellectual property and ownership issues are needed, especially as they relate to data sharing. In particular, the commercial exploitation of data or strains from less-wealthy countries must be addressed to account for concerns involving access to vaccines produced with their virus strains. Such agreements, it was noted, must simultaneously promote innovation and development internationally. Sequence data need to be widely shared while recognizing that intellectual property rights attached solely to the processes and products are created using this information.

Despite praise for the mounting success of U.S. efforts to promote public access to publicly funded data, it was questioned whether requirements to share data in other countries should or could be donor-driven (i.e., made a requirement of grants). The general perception was that there is significant merit to this approach, but that international donors and funding agencies may face resistance. While a culture change is needed to increase the acceptability of data sharing, it was recognized that it will take time and continued effort for such cultural shifts to occur worldwide. In the meantime, efforts to promote data sharing need to be initiated at regional levels.

While data-sharing improvements were considered necessary, participants cautioned that attention must be given to cost-benefit analyses of such efforts. Global surveillance systems can be extremely costly; therefore, it is imperative that these data structures maintain a sizable return on investment in terms of the public health impact they produce.

Participants discussed the concept of increased sharing of information being a "global good." What is accepted as a universal good by those in high-income versus low-income countries might differ depending on the needs and interests of different areas. With this in mind, policy responses need to carefully consider the issue of who benefits from increased data sharing.

There was broad discussion of the strategic and political considerations behind pandemic responses. These considerations included how to determine and balance the appropriate role of governments and international organizations, and a concern about overreach by these groups in trying to exert too much control. In particular, the role for international bodies such as the WHO and the World Organisation for Animal Health (OIE) in regulating or requiring data sharing was debated.

There was acknowledgment that research into antivirals needs to be supported as another tool in responding to pandemics. Antivirals were effectively used in response to PDM 2009 H1N1; therefore, expanding this tool for use in future outbreaks was considered an important goal to achieve.

The public health infrastructure for vaccine distribution is viewed as substandard in many parts of the world. This was illustrated by problems encountered when the U.S. attempted to donate 10% of its production of H1N1 vaccine to areas that could not afford to buy it. The countries that needed the vaccine the most did not have the capacity to distribute it and it took approximately 18 months to dispense the vaccine through the WHO. The continuing efforts to build infrastructure capacity in less-wealthy countries is crucial to ensuring that the benefits of improving infectious disease prediction and vaccine production are realized worldwide.

The public health infrastructure that was developed and strengthened to prepare for H5N1 and that successfully addressed PDM 2009 H1N1 cannot be allowed to decline. Efforts to increase and improve data sharing should build on this infrastructure. Additionally, there was a call for using the infrastructure constructed for responding to influenza as a platform for designing broader public health responses to other diseases.

Regulatory hurdles were identified as the biggest challenge to speeding the process of vaccine development. The importance of ensuring the safety and quality of vaccines, while allowing for expanded manufacturing capacity, was acknowledged as a critical set of parameters. However, regulators are reluctant to change their vaccine approval process. While no specific suggestions were provided as to how to change regulators' mindsets, convincing regulators to look at new technologies (e.g., process analytical technology) to decrease the time it takes to accept a vaccine as suitable for human use was considered imperative.

It was proposed that a One Flu approach should be expanded to include epidemiological investigations. To carry out effective risk assessments, epidemiologic data needs to be analyzed not only for specific outbreaks, but also to look across multiple-disease events.

The need to communicate the right messages to the public and to educate policy makers was emphasized. When the public is poorly informed, and misperceptions driven by inaccurate information in the public arena are not effectively corrected, efforts to mitigate infectious diseases are significantly undermined (e.g., H1N1 vaccine refusal in the U.S. that was prompted by concerns that the vaccine contained a fast-tracked adjuvant that causes serious side effects, despite the fact that the adjuvant had been licensed in Italy for a decade). The issue of risk was especially important to accurately convey to the public. Similarly, policy makers need to be educated regarding the health implications of their recommendations so that they make decisions based on credible science rather than uninformed media or public pressure.

Attention was drawn to the fact that global vaccine production heavily relies on manufacturing within India and China — two countries that possess approximately one-third of the world's population. Concern was voiced about the strategic implications of relying on vaccine production in these nations: in the event of a pandemic, domestic use requirements would limit the amount of vaccine available to other countries. It was questioned whether vaccine capacity should be developed in smaller countries, where enough vaccine could easily be produced to exceed the production country's population. Consequently, the surplus would be available for global distribution.

The Need for Expanded Global Efforts to Mitigate Viral Threats: Lessons from the HIV/AIDS Epidemic**

Robert C. Gallo, M.D.
Director, Institute of Human Virology,
University of Maryland School of Medicine
Director, Global Virus Network

Summary

There is a critical gap between current surveillance efforts and the implementation of clinical responses, caused primarily by the lack of international coordination for research on viral diseases and the shortage of medical virologists who will react once surveillance efforts uncover a problem. This gap jeopardizes the ability to deliver health services and threatens economies, supply chains, medical resources, and national and international security. Today, there is no single, recognized international organization empowered to speak with authority on all human viruses, though the need for such an organization has increased in recent decades. There are also serious deficiencies in training programs for research in medical virology, which threatens our future capacity to control viral epidemics. Finally, there is no mechanism to ensure that new viral threats are met with a sophisticated, international response to identify those viruses, develop new diagnostics, initiate the path to discovery of treatments or vaccines, and advise about the best mitigation strategies. To meet this need, the Global Virus Network (GVN) (http://www.ihv.org/programs/gvn.html), which is equipped with globally connected information technology enabling rapid communication between participants, has been formed (Nature, 2011). The GVN exemplifies the type of effort needed to mitigate the global threat of infectious diseases (see Figure 1).

Current realities

Despite the tremendous progress in the early years of HIV/AIDS, including the discovery of the first human retrovirus (HTLV-1) (1980), the discovery of HIV (1983–1984), the identification of HIV as the cause of AIDS (1984), and the development of the first systemic virus-specific therapy (1986), HIV/AIDS remains our number one viral problem today. Scientists agree that vaccination would be the best approach for long-term control and drug therapy remains best for slowing the disease.

There were great deficits in the global response to the HIV/AIDS pandemic, namely, that there were no medical virologists in positions of authority. Due to a lack of proper information technology (IT) infrastructure, the few available medical virologists were not equipped to communicate rapidly. Reflecting on the influenza epidemic of 1918 and the polio epidemic of the 1940s, mankind was unprepared to deal with such outbreaks. Today, we are well-equipped and have a wealth of knowledge from past mistakes. There is no excuse for failing to invest in the research, training, and global infrastructure needed to solve the current viral threats.

With respect to HIV/AIDS, one can argue that the United States Centers for Disease Control and Prevention (U.S. CDC) was responsible and prepared, and also performed early, critical, and accurate surveillance. However, the CDC does not have expertise in all human viruses. Indeed, at the onset of the AIDS epidemic, the CDC had no retrovirologists since such viruses were not considered to be human viruses. Moreover, the CDC only represents one country and is a function of the U.S. government. This often creates problems, and surely means that the CDC does not always speak out or freely counsel other governments.

Scientists who made key advances in virology came to the AIDS problem almost by chance during the early years. It was not their responsibility to initiate an effort to understand and combat HIV/AIDS. There was little sense that HIV represented a major threat and no organizations helped to prioritize and drive initial responses to this new disease. The global spread of viral threats has accelerated since that time. We no longer have the luxury of relying on serendipity to provide expertise needed to overcome significant threats to human health.

Scientific opportunities and challenges

In more recent years, the AIDS pandemic and the presence of new, visible funding (e.g., the Gates Foundation) have ensured that a significant number of active groups, organizations, and institutions are entering into the area of global infectious diseases. However, the chief problem remains and is getting worse. There is still no globally responsible organization to promote the engagement of medical virologists to combat new viral epidemics.

Another critical concern is an apparent decline in young people training for careers in virology. This may be due to the decline in young medical doctors going into basic research, reduced government support for infectious disease research, and public complacency about viral threats. An important consequence of our short-term memory about viral diseases is that we fail to support research and training programs needed to ensure the long-term supply of expert medical virologists. The extraordinary development of virus surveillance networks during the past 25 years produces a mountain of information, but without expert medical virologists, we are unprepared to grasp its importance and use it for developing disease mitigation strategies. An analogy can be used: lion hunters may be numerous and good at finding lions, but they need skilled experts who know how to deal with the lions once they have been found. Without a substantial and durable program for research and training, we remain ill-prepared in the face of constantly emerging viral threats.

We must also recognize that the absence of a single, authoritative, internationally recognized body of experts in medical virology opens the door to inappropriate and damaging responses to new viral diseases. This was exemplified by the economic losses and political embarrassment for China because of the Severe Acute Respiratory Syndrome (SARS) outbreak, which eventually had little more health impact than seasonal influenza. It is clear that screening efforts require the participation of a (nongovernmental) body of experts to formulate a rational response (See Figure 2 for other examples of global disasters).

The challenge is to fill the gaps in training, research, and policy-making that lie between virus surveillance efforts and health care delivery. Whereas agencies such as the CDC and the World Health Organization (WHO) provide surveillance networks, they do not have sufficient resources to address two critical questions: 1) What are the key aspects of viral threats which require new research? and 2) How can we train expert medical virologists to overcome the deficit and provide future scientists who recognize the imperative of international collaboration?

To meet the aforementioned challenges, in 2011, a group of leading virologists from 15 countries met and formed a nonprofit — the Global Virus Network (GVN). The GVN has set 10 goals to address these challenges: 1) an international base (see Figures 3 and 4); 2) freedom from political interests; 3) collaboration to advance our global knowledge; 4) training new virologists; 5) linkage to WHO; 6) advisory capacity to guide policy and share expertise on all classes of human viruses; 7) response to new threats; 8) virus discovery via research; 9) preparedness; and 10) global scientific exchange.

Policy makers should look upon the GVN goals as opportunities for policy actions. For example, in November 2010, Prime Minister Singh of India and U.S. President Obama signed a Memorandum of Understanding (MOU) creating a new Global Disease Detection (GDD) Center in New Delhi, which will facilitate preparedness against health threats such as pandemic influenza and other dangerous viruses (Padma, 2010). Several such GDD Centers have been established as part of a U.S. CDC program to enhance global capabilities, but they could be viewed as surveillance arms of the U.S. government. A good backup plan would be to link such centers as valuable nodes in the GVN, or another similar nongovernmental organization. New IT would make it possible to establish a global infrastructure to enable the rapid, secure exchange of information. Collecting, analyzing, reporting, and acting on this information would transform and enhance preparedness and would serve as a powerful, vital weapon to combat outbreaks.

Policy issues

- A recognized, sanctioned body of experts (e.g., the GVN) should be empowered to mitigate damage following early reports of viral outbreaks.
- Increase the stature and visibility of the GVN. Provide more opportunities for eminent scientists to become involved in multinational policy decisions.
- Facilitate liaisons between the GVN and other global bodies (organizations such as the Institute on Science for Global Policy [ISGP] could partner with the GVN as an advisory body and both should be chartered within the United Nations).
- Increase funding for global infectious disease organizations like the GVN to maintain collaborations, cross-fertilize, and share their expertise.
- Fund fellowship programs through governments, corporate partnerships, and nongovernmental organizations to train doctoral candidates in medical virology at the best virology institutes in the world.
- Global infectious disease organizations should be organized so each center is financed by its host country and a percentage of annual funding is "banked" by the organization for use in outbreak emergencies.
- Commit national and international funds to virus-discovery research.
- Establish IT infrastructure to improve global preparedness.

References

Nature. (March 3, 2011). Seven days: The news in brief — Viral response plan. Retrieved September 9, 2011, from http://www.nature.com/news/2011/110302/full/471010a.html

Padma, T. V. (2010, November 9). Obama's India visit generates science collaborations. Science and Development Network. Retrieved September 9, 2011, from http://www.scidev.net/en/news/obama-s-india-visit-generates-science-collaborations.html

** A policy position paper prepared for presentation at the conference on Emerging and Persistent Infectious Diseases (EPID): Focus on Mitigation convened by the Institute on Science for Global Policy (ISGP) Oct. 23–26, 2011, at the University of Edinburgh, Edinburgh, Scotland.

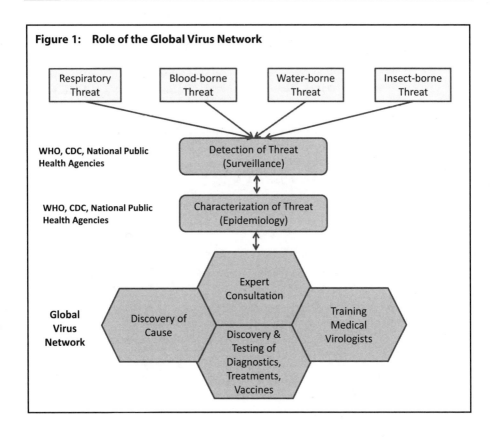

Figure 1:   Role of the Global Virus Network

Figure 2:   10 disasters that could have been averted, or at least diminished, if there had been a GVN

1. Polio pandemic.
2. Infection of thouisands of people in 1984 due to delays in accepting the HIV blood test. HIV pandemic.
3. Case of the Libyan nurses.
4. SARS debacle for China.
5. The "swine flu" pandemic.
6. The rise in global rabies incidence.
7. Dengue hemorrhagic fever expansion
8. Outbreaks due to anti-vaccine sentiment (e.g., measles, YF)
9. Slaughter of healthy animals containing "potentially dangerous" viruses.
10. Global rise in pox outbreaks.

Figure 3: Centers of Excellence in Virology Cover Expertise in All Known Viral Diseases

Centers	Retro viruses	Pox viruses	Herpes viruses	Respiratory viruses	DNA tumor viruses	Hemorrhagic fever viruses	Hepatis viruses	Enteric viruses	Neurotripic viruses
Africa S. African Natl Lab									
Australia Burnet Inst									
Canada Pacific Rim Consortium									
China Beijing, Shanghai									
Germany									
India									
Ireland									
Italy									
Israel Mideast Consortium									
Russia Baltic Consortium									
S. America									
Spain									
Sweden									
U.K. Glasgow Pirbright									
USA CO St. Univ; IHV Univ MD; Univ Mich.; Mt Sinai, NY; Gladstone; Univ Texas; J. Hopkins									

Figure 4: Global Virus Network Centers of Excellence in Virology

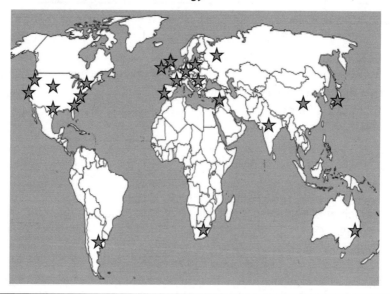

Debate Summary

The following summary is based on notes recorded by the ISGP staff during the not-for-attribution debate of the policy position paper prepared by Dr. Robert Gallo (see above). Dr. Gallo initiated the debate with a 5-minute statement of his views and then actively engaged the conference participants, including other authors, throughout the remainder of the 90-minute period. This Debate Summary represents the ISGP's best effort to accurately capture the comments offered and questions posed by all participants, as well as those responses made by Dr. Gallo. Given the not-for-attribution format of the debate, the views comprising this summary do not necessarily represent the views of Dr. Gallo, as evidenced by his policy position paper. Rather, it is, and should be read as, an overview of the areas of agreement and disagreement that emerged from all those participating in the critical debate.

Debate conclusions

- Because virology laboratories have generally become involved in infectious disease mitigation efforts by chance as opposed to through preplanned efforts, coordination of viral outbreak responses has traditionally been limited. Although the virology community has often responded well to outbreaks of new diseases (e.g., in the case of Severe Acute Respiratory Syndrome [SARS]), limited coordination means that a successful response cannot be guaranteed.
- Narrow scientific training within academic disciplines has presented obstacles in the training of scientists in general, and virologists specifically, since it does not prepare them to conduct research outside of their niches, or to adapt their work to address novel challenges. Additionally, increasing pressures within medical school curricula have limited opportunities for the training of clinician-scientists who could bring alternative medical perspectives to the field.
- The newly inaugurated Global Virus Network (GVN) is a vehicle through which improvements can be gained in the coordination of responses to viral outbreaks, as well as in the training for young virologists. At present, the virology community is falling short in both these pursuits.
- Given restricted funding environments, it is essential that the GVN effectively communicates its goals to overcome the generally short attention spans of the public and policy community.

- There is presently insufficient understanding within the scientific community about how to successfully carry out interdisciplinary projects. Current efforts are often characterized as too shallow because they frequently touch on many disciplines without going into depth in any of these areas.

Current realities

There was considerable debate concerning the current state of virology research around the globe. On one hand, a decrease in the number of physician-scientists since the 1980s may be responsible for a perceived decline in general biology research and, more specifically, virology research. This argument acknowledged the unique perspective and skill set that those with both medical and scientific training impart on research. However, medical training was not considered a prerequisite for being a successful researcher. It was further asserted that there is currently a considerable amount of high-quality virology research activity internationally and that other disciplines may be equally, if not more, in need of investment (e.g., epidemiology).

There has not been a designated agency or organization within the virology community to take the lead in the coordination of research and control efforts when new viruses emerge. Although the example of SARS was used to illustrate the successful mitigation of a pandemic by the virology community, serendipity may have been as influential as preplanned or coordinated efforts in controlling this disease. The suggestion that chance played such a significant role in the success of SARS mitigation nonetheless evoked the opinion that planning and preparedness for future viral pandemics require greater structure and cohesion.

The perceived decline in virology research was attributed in part to the growing interest in other scientific fields (e.g., genomics and synthetic biology). These perceptions have greatly contributed to the declining popularity of more traditional disciplines, such as virology. It was asserted that physicians, who previously comprised approximately one-third to one-half of all virologists, are increasingly eschewing research.

Problems emanate from medical training systems, which were perceived by some as being overly narrow and prescriptive. It was argued that current medical training (both pre- and post-qualification) does not equip doctors to become physician-scientists. An example cited was the system for training doctors in the United Kingdom, where the popularity of problem-based learning in medical schools means that doctors no longer have a sufficiently rigorous academic base on which to build a career in scientific research. Additionally, after qualification, clinical loads are so high that opportunities for scientific training are severely limited.

In many cases, medical training does not sufficiently expose students to tropical diseases. This was partially attributed to a decline in the practice of sending young doctors from more-wealthy countries to train abroad. As a result, doctors are unable to recognize diseases that are rare in their home countries (e.g., the U.K.), but common overseas. While there is presently an increased interest in global health among medical students, which has brought added attention to areas where infectious diseases are endemic, the constantly evolving and expanding medical curricula make it increasingly difficult to fit all relevant topics into student schedules. For example, epidemiology and virology are not always adequately emphasized within medical school curricula.

The recent creation of the GVN, which was established in part to address the aforementioned challenges, was a central theme of the debate. There was some uneasiness regarding the narrow focus of the GVN, given that it only applies to virology. Because research proposals that look at the differences between diseases tend to be favored over those that look at the similarities, scientists are rewarded for existing in "silos" and were viewed as uncomfortable working outside of their niches. The point was made that even a virologist who works on pox viruses would feel uncomfortable discussing issues related to other viruses such as HIV.

Scientific opportunities and challenges

The challenge of raising funds for the GVN, particularly at a time when budgets are stretched, was discussed. There was considerable debate over the significance of the US$10 million that will be required to fund the GVN annually. When the budgets of entire health departments are being cut due to a lack of funds, US$10 million will be considered a significant sum. However, this level of funding could easily be raised by a small number of philanthropists from the United States, Europe, India, and China. Additionally, while funding options are currently constrained by the difficult financial climate, improvements and innovations in technology are creating opportunities for progress that must be pursued.

Related to the issue of funding, there was considerable agreement that the current narrow focus of the GVN makes it a difficult concept to promote. This argument was predicated on the fact that, when resources are limited, it is difficult to convince people that an issue is relevant to them if there is no direct impact. For example, it was noted that it would be difficult to persuade the U.S. public to support an organization funding an overseas laboratory, even if that laboratory is undertaking invaluable virology research.

Successful promotion of the GVN was also thought to be hindered by constant shifts in the public and political popularity of various disciplines and causes (e.g., virology). It was accordingly argued that, as other disciplines (e.g., genomics and synthetic biology) gain popularity, maintaining a strong focus on virology research becomes challenging. This problem was compounded by the fact that public awareness of and interest in science is generally very low. Indeed, it was suggested that maintaining long-term support for the GVN would necessitate transformations in the way that society relates to science. As part of this, it was considered the responsibility of the scientific community to convince the public of the value of science. In the shorter term, films like "Contagion" could be used as a vehicle to promote awareness and encourage support.

Challenges related to the "siloization" or "stove piping" of the different disciplines working on infectious diseases were extensively discussed. Concern was raised about siloization in the field of virology itself, as well as across infectious disease research more generally. Although there are many positive aspects of the trend toward narrow specializations in science, such restricted foci are problematic for infectious disease preparedness. For example, virologists tend to be so narrowly focused within their discipline (e.g., pox virology, HIV) that they are rarely prepared to address major viral outbreaks when they occur, particularly if the virus does not fit within commonly recognized patterns.

The challenge of promoting general research, which would give virologists an improved, broader skill set when dealing with new and emerging viruses, was recognized as requiring greater attention. There was consensus that the development of a virology training program within the GVN could provide a means to mitigate this specialization problem. Young virologists could spend six months training in three different centers or laboratories (18 months total) that focus on distinct subsets of virology, followed by the writing of a thesis, for which they would receive a certificate from the GVN. Such a training program would ensure that virologists have a greater breadth of experience than is currently the case, thereby considerably strengthening the pool of virology researchers. A warning was sounded, however, that even if such training opportunities were to be developed, it is extremely difficult to maintain such general skills across a career.

The considerable difficulties related to the establishment of broader interdisciplinary research programs were also discussed. It was suggested that interdisciplinary research is difficult to execute and fund due to widespread perceptions that such studies garner only superficial results. Since it is exceptionally difficult to create strong interdisciplinary links while simultaneously fostering the specific aims of each individual discipline, it was concluded that depth of understanding is sacrificed as a consequence. For example, a recent call by a major funding agency for research projects that would study the ecology, environment, and sociology of emerging infections failed to fund any of the submitted research proposals because none were deemed to be strong enough in all of the disciplinary areas they covered. Research has been published on how best to develop, fund, and evaluate interdisciplinary studies, but the advice is rarely heeded. Additionally, it takes very specific skill sets to successfully run interdisciplinary projects, which the majority of specialists either do not have or recognize as a priority.

Concern was raised that the GVN would do little to break down barriers between disciplines. However, those who did not feel that this was either its purpose or a priority countered that the GVN would fill a much-needed niche in pure virology expertise, which is essential for establishing a scientific base that can be drawn on when new diseases emerge. Moreover, if the scope of the GVN was expanded, it would be difficult to discern where to draw the line in defining its purpose.

Because there are currently no designated virologists to take the lead when new viruses emerge, the ability of the public health community to coordinate and launch effective responses against viral emergence was thought to be a considerable challenge. Although prior responses to some viruses (e.g., SARS) have been successful, it was agreed that many of these positive outcomes were largely due to decisions being made haphazardly rather than a well-coordinated effort. The recently inaugurated GVN could fill a critical gap by being the first in line to provide expertise and advice when a virus emerges. The establishment of the GVN as a key advisory organization could also provide a significant opportunity to improve public health responses to emerging viruses. Based on the characteristics of an emerging virus, the GVN would be able to identify which virology laboratories are best equipped to assist in coordinating a response. Members of the GVN would be able to forge and utilize links between virology laboratories to ensure that the coordination is effective. While there was general agreement that the GVN offers important opportunities for improved planning and preparedness in the face of an epidemic, it was argued that the organization will only be truly successful in this regard if it works in conjunction with other agencies.

Three of the most significant viral outbreaks — HIV, influenza, and SARS — all mutated to jump the species barrier from animals into humans. There was some disagreement over the state of funding for veterinary research related to the movement of viruses across species. Despite the animal origins of many viruses, funding and provisions for veterinary virology research generally fall far short of what is available for human virology research (particularly in less-affluent countries). The tremendous contribution that veterinary virologists have made to the advancement of human health was noted, and it was suggested that a challenge for the GVN lies in ensuring that veterinary virology is adequately integrated into its work.

Policy issues

Concern was expressed regarding the gulf between scientific understanding and policy priorities. In a climate where policy is made not by "rational" processes, but by political objectives, it can be difficult to determine whether the outcome of any policy decision will be positive or negative from a scientific perspective. The efforts to raise funds and garner interest for the GVN must take this political reality into account.

A significant portion of the debate centered on the potential difficulty of raising money for the GVN. It was argued that money is not an impediment because the estimated cost of running the GVN (US$10 million annually) could be easily met by philanthropists. By contrast, it was noted that this sum could be difficult to raise in the current economic climate, and equally difficult to sustain over time. It was noted that the GVN will likely need to be able to show a return on investment to maintain funding. To counterbalance both global economic concerns and shifting scientific interests away from virology (e.g., toward genomics), the need for a permanent and sustainable funding structure was made clear. Thus, a significant policy issue for the GVN to consider is the running of a coherent communications campaign that would galvanize support from outside the virology community and bolster funding.

An alternate model for increasing financial investment in virology was suggested, whereby funding agencies are proactive in assessing a problem and identifying which individuals or research groups might be able to solve it. An alternative view, strongly held, was that an over-reliance on funding agencies is undesirable since it would mean that the success of organizations such as the GVN would rise and fall based on public and political whim as opposed to scientific necessity.

Increased funding to the GVN might also have the unintended effect of increasing siloization and stove piping. Hypothetically, the viral focus of the GVN might result in more money being funneled into narrow niches and distinct programs, as opposed to cross-disciplinary activities or other broad areas (e.g., public health infrastructure). However, the relatively small amount of money needed for the GVN would not require funds being siphoned off from elsewhere, particularly if it is raised through philanthropy.

The geographical distribution of where training and resources are allocated was debated. It was argued that the global economy will be increasingly centered on the Indian Ocean region; therefore, networks such as the GVN cannot be successful if they primarily focus on Europe and the U.S. Young scientists from Asia need to be engaged in networks like the GVN, and training opportunities and resources need to be directed to them. Countries such as India are becoming increasingly involved in the GVN, though local issues can sometimes hinder their involvement.

The question of which countries the GVN should engage with was also raised. It was noted that relationships are already being forged with Vietnam, the Caribbean, and a number of countries in Africa. However, it was emphasized that the GVN should not be too ambitious too fast regarding the number of countries it interacts with, and also that it should only link to institutions with outstanding virology programs.

It was considered critical for current systems of training scientists to be reviewed and restructured. Since government priorities have resulted in many students being trained to follow "black and white" protocols, many are unable to take a nuanced approach to scientific research. It was deemed crucial that a new cadre of students, comfortable with cross-disciplinary research, and knowledgeable about the diseases that affect both more- and less-wealthy countries, be nurtured through training. The GVN could be an ideal organization to advocate for improvements in this area.

Concern was voiced regarding a proposal to charter the GVN to the United Nations (UN). It was argued that this would be a complicated and laborious process that would not reap benefits for the GVN. Establishing the GVN as a professional, international association would carry more weight and influence than being chartered to the UN. It is more important for the GVN to gain significant recognition than for it to become chartered to an international organization.

The GVN can be most effective if it works in collaboration both with international organizations (e.g., the World Health Organization [WHO]) and governmental organizations (e.g., the U.S. Centers for Disease Control and Prevention [CDC]). It was acknowledged, however, that such partnerships need to be tempered with a level of independence since it was considered important for the GVN, as an independent body, to be able to speak out on sensitive issues in a way that a governmental organization cannot. The case of the Bulgarian nurses (who were accused in 1998 of deliberately infecting Libyan children with HIV) was provided as an example of the discrepancy between governments and independent organizations in their ability to express a particular stance. While the CDC was unable to speak in the nurses' defense, the GVN would have been able to do so had it existed at that time. For this reason, informal links, rather than "special relationships" between the GVN and governmental bodies, were advocated.

Communicating Risk in the Age of Information Plenty: Implications for Policy and Practice of Emerging and Persistent Infectious Diseases (EPID)**

Kasisomayajula "Vish" Viswanath, Ph.D.
Associate Professor, Harvard School of Public Health
Associate Professor, Dana-Farber Cancer Institute
Faculty Director, Health Communication Core,
Dana-Farber/Harvard Cancer Center

Summary

Policy makers and public health practitioners are wrestling with how to communicate and mitigate risks of infectious diseases through various mechanisms at the national level (e.g., country governments), as well as the transnational level (e.g., the World Health Organization [WHO]). The 20th century-designed communication planning, however, is confronting a 21st century reality — a revolution in communication and information technologies with significant consequences for Emerging and Persistent Infectious Diseases (EPID). The consequences of this revolution include: the generation of a large amount of information and transmission of this information at speeds that allow little control over how it is interpreted by different groups; difficulty among institutions and social groups in assessing and communicating risk accurately; and widening communication inequalities among individuals, groups, and nations. To address current challenges in communicating about disease risks, a new transnational information and communication "architecture," with the following four core elements, is needed: (1) development and maintenance of capacity to assess, interpret, and communicate risks as expeditiously as possible; (2) continuous surveillance of the information environment to monitor how risk communication about EPID is occurring, to facilitate quick and prompt action; (3) promotion of policies and practices that mitigate the inequalities in communication of risk; and (4) continued research to develop evidence-based risk communication strategies.

Current realities

The ways in which infectious disease risk information fares, once it enters the public arena, is of primary concern. This process may be examined under three broad areas: the generation (origin) of information, the public arena, and the reception and effects of risk communications.

Generation of risk information. It is now widely recognized that communication is a critical part of any risk management strategy and in contemporary societies, determining how and what to communicate to the public is a complex process. To make decisions regarding both the timing and content of risk communication, coordination and communication among different agencies is necessary. However, the decisions usually are made in a complex environment where authority may be spread over different agencies and the political, social, and cultural context of the audience varies widely. From a communication perspective, questions may include mundane issues such as who decides to take the lead on communication, what policies and procedures are in place, and when and how to release the information. More critical and complicated decisions involve how the information is framed and communicated to diverse audiences whose social, cultural, and economic backgrounds may vary considerably. It is also critical to consider the communication infrastructure of a given country, both in terms of trained professional communicators and the penetration of different media to reach different publics.

The public arena. The degree of control exercised by the authorities over risk communication messages is immediately challenged and seized once it enters the public arena. As a result, the information environment on EPID is possibly more complex than it has ever been, raising questions about how and what to communicate about risk. Three broad groups, with varying degrees of specialization, expertise, and resources, influence how the information is further diffused to the public: journalists, the entertainment media, and interest groups.

One, journalists are important gatekeepers between the authorities and the public. On a positive note, since reporters use communications from authorities to generate many story ideas (e.g., press releases and press conferences), sometimes these messages are included almost verbatim in the news stories. On the other hand, journalists are under deadline pressure, prefer clear story lines, and work under limitations of space and time. In addition, few journalists have a formal background in science or medicine, which could have positive or negative consequences for the accurate communication of risk information. Two, a developing body of work is documenting the clear and often powerful effects of entertainment media on risk-related behaviors such as tobacco use, obesity, risky sex, and violence. Little, however, is known about the role of popular culture and entertainment media in communication and interpretation of the risks of EPID and their mitigation. Three, the revolution in Information and Communication

Technologies (ICTs) is upending the way people and institutions generate information, communicate, and interact with each other. The Internet has successfully led to the steady erosion of the oligopoly of conventional media over the generation and dissemination of information. "User-generated" content allows risk information to be interpreted by anyone, which is actually done by millions of bloggers and microbloggers through social media. Bloggers and stakeholders may be seen as having credibility, expertise, and ideologies (or even kookiness). They offer multiple interpretations of "facts" about infectious diseases and ways to "mitigate" them, potentially sowing seeds of confusion.

Reception and effects of risk communication. This relates to how the ways that audiences encounter risk information influences their knowledge, attitudes, and behaviors with regard to EPID and efforts to mitigate EPID. Audiences may encounter risk information (e.g., on avian flu) in two ways. The most common encounter may be characterized as "incidental exposure" — information obtained through routine use of media for news or entertainment (e.g., television, newspapers or magazines, Internet, and radio). In addition, social networks are an important source of exposure and interpretation. Audiences also encounter risk information when actively seeking information either for themselves or for others, especially when facing a threat of any kind.

A variety of personality, individual, cultural, and social factors influence exposure, seeking, and subsequent risk communication effects. Of note, at the individual level, people's perceptions of the safety of mitigating actions, such as vaccines, influence whether they take action. Trust in authorities is also a critical determinant of whether people follow and act on information. Both personal susceptibility as well as severity of the threat may also influence how they receive and act on information. The role of social class is of enormous importance as a factor in influencing exposure, understanding, and acting on risk information — a phenomenon characterized as communication inequalities. It is now well established that social class (usually measured as schooling) plays a significant role in what kind of channels people access and use, as well as the degree to which they can process that information and act on it. In general, people who are relatively poor are less likely to use channels such as the Internet and print media, and have difficulty in processing the information and limited capacity to act on it. Numeracy, the ability to interpret quantitative information, is also strongly associated with class. Communication inequalities are a worldwide phenomenon, both among individuals and nations, with profound implications for communication of risk about EPID.

Scientific opportunities and challenges

Related to the 21st century information environment, five scientific challenges and opportunities are especially critical: (1) Information on EPID is complex, competing with other topics; this raises questions about how to attract and maintain the attention of the audience; (2) How are communications about risks of EPID tracked and how can misinterpretations be countered? No known models of information surveillance systems exist at this point; (3) It is widely accepted that those who are among the poor, and in lower- and middle-income nations, are at great risk of EPID and its consequences compared with those who are well off and in wealthier nations. By extension, the specific effects of culture and class on EPID risk information remain to be explored; (4) In a related vein, we need more scientific evidence on what role different media, genres, and formats play in communicating about the risks of EPID and with what consequences; (5) Lastly, ICTs, particularly mobile media, offer an enormous potential to reach people who have been bypassed by earlier communication revolutions. Mobile technologies and related software, such as text messaging, in combination with social media, could be exploited to bridge inequalities and disparities, providing a historic opportunity. Their value remains an empirical question.

Policy issues

Recommendations for science, policy, and practice in the context of EPID include:

- **Development of a transnational risk information and communication architecture that involves national and international agencies.** With the development of ICTs, there are many opportunities to tap the software of the cyber infrastructure to track, analyze, and disseminate risk information about EPID. Public-private partnerships, where the private sector develops the technologies and the public sector fields and tests them, should be created. Optimally, an organization such as WHO should take the lead in association with other agencies such as the International Telecommunication Union (ITU) and the private sector.
- **Investment in human capital to assess, interpret, and communicate risks of EPID as expeditiously as possible.** Given the pace of movement and the rapidity with which infectious diseases and information are spread, it is critical that countries have capacity in the form of risk communicators (e.g., Public Information Officers) within their health agencies. While multilateral organizations, such as the World Bank or WHO, can provide

the technical assistance and lead training efforts, much of the action is likely to occur within the governments of the countries themselves.

- **Investment in the science, dissemination, and implementation of evidence-based risk communication strategies.** Building scientific capacity for basic research in risk communication science is in the purview of a variety of sectors. Research institutions and universities should take the lead here with support from the private sector and government.

- **Promotion of access to ICT to mitigate inequalities in risk communication.** Given the enormous inequalities in communication, even the most thoughtful risk communication strategy is unlikely to result in effective mitigation. National governments should recognize the value of access to ICT, and offer subsidies where necessary to promote access.

References

Lipkus, I. M. (2007). Numeric, verbal, and visual formats of conveying health risks: Suggested best practices and future recommendations. Medical Decision Making, 27(5), 696–713.

Visschers, V. H., Meertens, R. M., Passchier, W. W., & de Vries, N. N. (2009). Probability information in risk communication: A review of the research literature. Risk Analysis, 29(2), 267–287.

Viswanath K. Public communications and its role in reducing and eliminating health disparities. In: Thomson GE, Mitchell F, Williams MB, editors. Examining the health disparities research plan of the National Institutes of Health: Unfinished business. Washington (DC): Institute of Medicine; 2006. p. 215–253.

*** A policy position paper prepared for presentation at the conference on Emerging and Persistent Infectious Diseases (EPID): Focus on Mitigation convened by the Institute on Science for Global Policy (ISGP) Oct. 23–26, 2011, at the University of Edinburgh, Edinburgh, Scotland.*

Debate Summary

The following summary is based on notes recorded by the ISGP staff during the not-for-attribution debate of the policy position paper prepared by Prof. Kasisomayajula "Vish" Viswanath (see above). Prof. Viswanath initiated the debate with a 5-minute statement of his views and then actively engaged the conference participants, including other authors, throughout the remainder of the 90-minute period. This Debate Summary represents the ISGP's best effort to accurately capture the comments offered and questions posed by all participants, as well as those responses made by Prof. Viswanath. Given the not-for-attribution format of the debate, the views comprising this summary do not necessarily represent the views of Prof. Viswanath, as evidenced by his policy position paper. Rather, it is, and should be read as, an overview of the areas of agreement and disagreement that emerged from all those participating in the critical debate.

Debate conclusions

- As the dissemination of and access to disease information expands, the health and science communities are increasingly losing control over how such information is interpreted. Consequently, messages about health issues from credible scientists and agencies are often confused by inaccurate, incomplete, and competing information from diverse sources. Thus, the 21st century information and technology environment has complicated efforts to effectively communicate a credible understanding of disease risk to the public and has made it difficult for individuals to distinguish fact from opinion, to accurately identify their risk, and to decide which health recommendations to follow.

- The existence of diverse types of "publics" (also known as "communities of interpretation") ensures that a "one size fits all" approach to communication cannot be effectively employed to craft and deliver messages concerning health risks, even for the same disease. To strengthen compliance with interventions, tailored messages from multiple sources, all perceived by these publics to be credible and trusted, must be developed that reflect localized values, beliefs, concerns, perceptions of risk, customs, and agendas.

- To improve the effectiveness of risk messaging during a crisis, evidence-based risk communication needs to be delivered proactively. To properly shape this type of communication for the public, such messages must consider (i) the information content itself, (ii) how the content is presented as numbers, facts, and/or stories, and (iii) the dissemination channels to be used, including mobile phones, Internet, and television and film.

- Relationships among the scientific community, policy makers, and the media need to be significantly improved to facilitate the presentation of scientific evidence in ways that accurately inform the public. Priority needs to be given to providing training in risk communication to all scientists, public health professionals, and government representatives who may be responsible for risk assessments to the public concerning diseases outbreaks. To be effective, communication strategies need to be proactively developed and ready for implementation during an actual event. Moreover, relationships with trusted societal leaders and the media must be established in advance by cultivating individuals who can help galvanize these groups if events demand coordinated messaging.

Current realities

It was asserted that current risk communication policies and practices, which were primarily designed in and for the 20th century, are largely ineffective in the 21st century information and technology environment. As part of a discussion of specific characteristics of current information technology and practices, it was agreed that an enormous amount of health and science information is now distributed to the public and that such information is obtained from a much broader array of sources than in the past. This was contrasted with the pre-21st century environment where a small number of entities were able to distribute information in a careful, controlled, and presumably accurate way. As information dissemination and access expands, the health and science communities are increasingly losing control over how information is interpreted. Facts about disease risks and their impact on human health are now interpreted and reinterpreted in the public arena. Consequently, messages about health from credible scientists and agencies are often being contradicted, overshadowed and/or ignored by sources using misinformation or having an incomplete understanding of the data available.

While the "democratization of information" (i.e., the increasing number of entities with control over the dissemination of information, accurate or inaccurate) was lauded for enhancing people's access to knowledge, it was widely recognized that the decentralization of information sources has simultaneously complicated efforts to accurately and effectively communicate risk. It was noted that people do not always pay attention to the topics prioritized by the scientific and policy communities due to the large volume of information that continually competes for their attention. The communication of accurate information about disease risks has become increasingly difficult, but there was agreement that the recognizable hurdles are not insurmountable.

Certain organizations, some of which remain trusted by the public, were recognized as undermining the influence of credible scientific and technological understanding by publicizing inaccurate or distorted information. Such organizations can impede the ability of credible scientists to shape and transmit useful messages and thus significantly influence the public's perceptions of risk, and alter individuals' willingness to comply with advice concerning interventions. These conflicting messages were illustrated by specific examples, including the historical efforts by certain groups to frame genetically modified (GM) technology in a negative light and the resultant damage to the public's perceptions of the food produced by GM technology.

Despite the perceived overabundance of information disseminated to the public, it was recognized that certain sources (e.g., specific Web sites and television stations) are more trusted than others to provide accurate information. The public's assessment of the credibility of information is greatly shaped by an individual's "filters," which include factors such as age, culture, and education. Younger generations, known as "millenials," have "looser" filters (i.e., they are less skeptical about information and its sources and are more comfortable with ambiguous facts and a lack of certitude). Looser filters among younger populations were highlighted as a current source of concern.

There was some disagreement about the role of journalists in conveying risk information. It was noted that in recent years journalists have become less important as gatekeepers and communicators of information in general. While the influence of mainstream media is eroding, research shows that journalists remain critical information sources about human health issues. However, it is clear that given the generally limited scientific backgrounds of most journalists, this community remains constrained in its ability to accurately communicate scientific information to the public.

It was agreed that there are diverse publics, defined by their divergent customs, concerns, socioeconomic backgrounds, and geographic locations. These factors affect their respective perceptions of the causes and risks of disease. As a result, individuals within these publics comply differently to advice concerning interventions. Such concerns (e.g., vaccine risks) may vary both between and within countries.

Differences between the concepts of communication content, format, and platforms were discussed. Content was described as the actual information, or message, that is provided. Format was characterized as the presentation of the content (e.g., numbers, facts, and/or stories). Platforms were defined as the channels through which such messages are disseminated (e.g., mobile phones, Internet, television/film, social media, and newspapers). Each one of these communication components can alter the effectiveness of infectious disease messaging.

It was acknowledged that compliance with interventions designed to prevent the spread of infectious diseases is sometimes fueled by factors that are unrelated to public health efforts (including communication), but which nevertheless impact risk perception. A country-specific example was provided where the death of a celebrity, due to the H1N1 strain of influenza, changed the public's perception of risk and as a result, led to increased vaccine uptake.

While the information revolution has led to widespread communication technologies, research has shown that the effects on and benefits within given communities have been unequal depending on socioeconomic and geographic factors. Although many believe everyone has equal access to information in a given geographical region, it is evident that access to and benefits from advanced communication technologies disproportionately benefit those of higher socioeconomic status. In addition to having the information available to them, it is clear that the degree to which individuals process and utilize information can reflect their respective levels of literacy and social experience. Even those who have the knowledge to act on information often encounter limiting social and physical barriers, both within and between countries.

Scientific opportunities and challenges

The most significant challenge to accurate risk communication was seen as the erosion of control in how information is disseminated, which has made it difficult for the public to distinguish fact from opinion, accurately perceive risk, and decide which health recommendations to follow. The question was raised regarding how much information members of the public can be expected to acquire or understand, given that they are constantly flooded with facts and recommendations.

Much of the discussion focused on the most effective ways to communicate risk in light of the challenges associated with recent transformations in information technology and the role of social networking. It was argued that scientific research on public opinion and communications should be employed to articulate, frame, and define issues that have public health benefit. In realms outside of public health, the science of public opinion and communications is being used to challenge, influence, and redirect the public agenda. The importance of paying attention to nuances in public opinion research, and staying informed as public opinion and communication science evolves, was underscored. While existing research already provides some information about effective, alternative ways of communicating risk, further investigation was called for to strengthen the evidence base.

The unique epidemiology of infectious disease has implications for risk communication. Changes in disease incidence were highlighted as a prominent instigator of shifts in risk perception and decision-making. For example, during times of crisis, the public can be more easily convinced to comply with interventions, such as vaccinations. However, with so much competing information, members of the public typically do not pay attention to their risk of disease unless there is an emergency. In some cases, where the risk of the intervention outweighs the risk of disease, the risk calculus favors non-compliance causing rational actors to not comply. To sustain the public good and avoid disease proliferation and/or re-emergence, it was seen as imperative to convince the public to accept the risks associated with interventions. Yet, effectively communicating risk/benefit tradeoffs to the public remains a major societal and governmental challenge.

There was general consensus that a "one size fits all" approach cannot be employed for crafting and delivering messages concerning public health, even for the same disease. Researchers need to identify the values, beliefs, concerns, perceptions of risk, customs, and agendas of specific communities (i.e., different "publics") as prerequisites to developing tailored, effective messages. Such approaches must address specific geographic, demographic and/or cultural groups and even groups with specific agendas (e.g., politicians, reporters, professional societies, patient advocacy groups). For example, millenials' adeptness at science and technology can be harnessed to improve outreach to this group. It would be helpful for public health communication efforts to follow the example of the private sector where success in selling products is often based on a detailed knowledge of their customers.

Perceived credibility was identified as a critical determinant of where people seek the information. In the recent case of H1N1, a national study showed that in the United States, local television news was the first source of information for most people. It was generally agreed that when risk information is not conveyed through trusted community sources, compliance can be significantly jeopardized. The central question, therefore, is how policy makers identify specific trusted sources when there are so many diverse characteristics. It was noted that there is a relatively good body of existing research that helps to identify the trusted, credible sources for communications with different publics. Cooperation with such sources is needed to properly tailor the messaging to these specific publics.

Because people rely on and trust different sources, it was agreed that the public's response to messaging would be greatly improved by communication efforts that employ multiple outlets to relay information. It was noted that certain channels, which are known to be effective, are currently underutilized. This was illustrated by the example of health care workers, who are often overlooked as an important conduit for communicating risk messages. There was a call for determining how to engage health care workers and provide them with the information they need to deliver key messages.

Coordinating the timing of risk communication is also important. There was general agreement that educating the public about risk in advance of a crisis is difficult, but that messages developed before a crisis based on sound risk communication principles can be employed with great effect as soon as an emergency occurs. It was cautioned that the scientific community's understanding of health threats evolves as new research results become available. If the message changes after it is initially conveyed to the public, scientists' credibility may be questioned. Reminding the public that credible scientific understanding is continuously evolving is a challenging but important element in maintaining public confidence.

Opportunities exist for currently available technologies to be further utilized in targeting and customizing risk communication. Examples were provided where successful interventions employed social networking and mobile technologies. Social media, for instance, has been implemented to enhance vaccine distribution efforts in the U.S. Specifically, local health departments have used Twitter and other social networking technologies to inform parents about vaccine availability at specific locations, wait times, and other relevant details. Cellular phone technology has also been used in the U.S. to send pregnant women informative text messages during different stages of pregnancy. While technology is not universally accessible, it was noted that technology is being increasingly employed in less-wealthy countries for public health purposes.

Information surveillance — whereby scientists can identify "who" is tracking "what," as well as which pieces of information are drawing people's attention at any given moment — was identified as an important mechanism that can be used for improving risk communications. An information surveillance environment would allow the public health community to understand people's evolving concerns and intervene appropriately.

Policy issues

While it was acknowledged that there are benefits to the democratization of information, much of the discussion focused on the role of policy makers in controlling information within an environment where credible scientists are being drowned out by vast amounts of misinformation in the public domain. There was significant discussion and disagreement over how policy makers can and should correct misperceptions about risk. Throughout the debate, the measles, mumps, and rubella (MMR) vaccine was used as an example where erroneous information regarding negative consequences (e.g., a false link to autism) has led to decreased compliance with public health intervention that has proven benefits. It was noted that celebrity spokespeople have played roles in spreading misinformation, and that the public health community and scientists have thus far not held people liable for spreading incorrect information. To resolve this problem, it was contended that efforts should be made to discredit these groups publicly.

A large portion of the discussion focused on which strategies should be used to promote public health messages and correct information misperceptions, with questions raised about the moral and ethical use of some strategies. Proactive risk communication may require damage control, including attacking sites that are producing and spreading false or misleading misinformation. There was significant disagreement concerning whether government agencies and others can "manipulate" Web-based information for the benefit of the public's health. Search Engine Optimization (SEO), often used by private industries to ensure that their information rises to the top of Internet searches, was recommended as one potential way to counter misinformation. It was asserted that public health agencies are reticent to use the types of calculated methods that are commonly employed by commercial firms and companies, but this viewpoint was countered by those who felt that these actions should not be viewed as manipulation. Rather, it was argued, such strategies should be considered an act of social responsibility, which is necessary to ensure that the public receives needed information.

As part of the discussion on determining which tactics policy makers and public health officials should consider using to convey accurate public health information, it was cautioned that there is a danger in viewing all scientists as being "credible." Several historical examples of the scientific community engaging in unethical practices (e.g., the Tuskegee experiments) were discussed and it was also noted that some scientists have promoted incorrect information (e.g., those who denied the relationship between HIV and AIDS). It was seen as important to provide the public with health science information using a judicious approach that accurately reflects the degree of uncertainty associated with any specific recommendation.

An emerging body of work investigating the effectiveness of different formats for communicating information can, and should, be used to shape how public health messages are delivered. For instance, individuals in the public arena are not as receptive to messages focused solely on facts, numbers, and probabilities because they are often not comfortable with this type of information. Entertainment and human-oriented news stories were identified as more successful messaging formats; scientific evidence is more rapidly absorbed when presented in the form of stories that relate to individuals because they are likely to capture the public's attention and people are not as likely to argue with information presented as a narrative.

Framing the public health message in a manner that resonates with the public was seen as especially critical, given that many sources regularly compete for attention. Utilizing the skills of risk analysis experts would strengthen how communication content is shaped. In addition, because studies have demonstrated that perception is a stronger determinant of behavior than actual risk, it was also considered important for message content to influence risk perception. It was advised that the two components of risk perception — severity and susceptibility — should be carefully addressed within communications efforts.

The need to improve the relationships among the scientific community, policy makers, and the media was strongly endorsed. An existing model was described and lauded for its effectiveness in bringing together scientists and the media. In this model, a group of editors with different news organizations is available to discuss publishing articles written by scientists. There was a call for such models to be replicated to facilitate the presentation of scientific evidence in ways that engage the general public.

It was widely agreed that science and medical graduates, public health professionals, policy makers, and all prospective crisis spokespeople need to be trained in risk and media communication. Such training is becoming more commonplace. For example, several important international funders currently provide communication training to grant and fellowship holders, and universities are increasingly focused on communication training. However, it was agreed that more work is needed in the realm of training, such as government agencies mandating communication training as a requirement for grant funding. There was also a call for ensuring that governmental and intergovernmental organizations (e.g., the U.S. Centers for Disease Control and Prevention, the World Health Organization, and the United Nations) employ staff members who are skilled at communicating and developing relationships with the media.

The importance of determining how to obtain higher vaccination compliance was discussed. It was argued that legislation can help overcome the barriers associated with public perceptions and changing realities (e.g., when the risks of vaccination outweigh the benefits). The general success of the U.S. approach, in which immunizations are mandated as a prerequisite to school attendance, was noted. Surprise was expressed that this approach has not been adopted more widely worldwide.

Planning for Pandemics: The Formulation of Policy**

Roy Anderson, F.R.S., F.Med.Sci.
Chair of Infectious Disease Epidemiology,
Department of Infectious Disease Epidemiology,
Faculty of Medicine, Imperial College London

Summary

The historical and epidemiological literature abounds with accounts of infectious disease epidemics and of the concomitant effects on population abundance, social organization and the unfolding pattern of historical events. Epidemics have long been a source of fear and fascination in human societies, but it is only in comparatively recent times that their origins and patterns have begun to yield their secrets through scientific study.

Current realities

The World Health Organization (WHO) has guidelines for defining a pandemic and on epidemic and pandemic alert and response (WHO, 2009). These guidelines are under revision following the 2009 H1N1 pandemic (PDM 2009 H1N1), in which guidance was largely based on patterns of spread from country to country, rather than spread and pathogenicity combined. Some novel infectious agents spread worldwide, but induce little impact on human health (e.g., many common cold viruses), whereas others are highly virulent (e.g., Severe Acute Respiratory Syndrome [SARS]).

Methods of analysis and interpretation for epidemics have advanced rapidly in recent years with many mathematical and computational tools available to predict spread, control impact, and define an optimal mitigation intervention package based on the available tools.

The SARS epidemic was handled well by the international community and controlled rapidly as a consequence. However, for various biological and epidemiological reasons, this was an easy pathogen to control by simple public health measures such as quarantine and patient isolation. Pathogens like influenza A are much more difficult to control due to rapid spread and short generation times (i.e., a few days). An error in handling the recent H1N1 pandemic was a failure to rapidly establish (by serological studies) the case fatality and serious morbidity rates for the new viral strain. If the fact that these were no higher than a typical seasonal influenza strain had been understood in a timely manner, the global response may have differed greatly to that which was put in place.

Scientific opportunities and challenges

The study of epidemic pattern and disease control has advanced in the past few decades from observation, through theory, to experiment and prediction. Increasingly, the concepts of evolution are embedded in the analysis of epidemics and this is especially so for pandemics of the influenza viruses. An increasing understanding of process and pattern in the emergence of pandemics has concomitantly resulted in better planning and policy formulation. Retrospective analysis of both the recent PDM 2009 H1N1 influenza epidemic and the preceding problem of SARS, which emerged in 2003, provides policy makers with guidance on what went well and what could be improved upon.

Early indications of a new pathogen's emergence are based on reports of unusual clusters of morbidity and mortality in space and time. Collation of such reports in real time is still primitive in the international practice of public health compared with other sectors such as meteorology, oceanography, and financial services. Even within very rich countries, digital data capture in real time is still an ambition rather than a reality. Current surveillance is based on Web-based searches of the media, in as wide a range of countries as possible, using algorithms that identify reports of unusual morbidity and mortality.

Once the clusters of disease cases are believed to be caused by an infectious agent, the key tasks are many and varied. These are summarized in Box 1. Identification and the demonstration of Koch's postulates (four criteria for establishing whether a specific organism is the cause of a particular disease) is the starting point and other tasks can be initiated simultaneously. The SARS pandemic well illustrated the power of international collaboration, which was demonstrated by the combined efforts of WHO, existing university linkages, and professional bodies.

Mathematical and computational tools, which are more akin to the methods employed in the physical and engineering sciences, have had slow uptake in many public health and medical circles. Many still rely on a consensus arising from verbal discussions in advisory committees rather than on quantitative analysis.

At the earliest stages of the emergence of a novel agent, focus is typically on diagnosis and treatment. Treatment may not be an option for some time (e.g., perhaps six months at a minimum for a vaccine and longer for a drug) given the development delays in producing drugs and vaccines even in an emergency. Often forgotten is the need to measure key epidemiological variables that determine rates of spread, impact of possible public health interventions (e.g., quarantine), and the possible time scale of global spread. For the SARS virus responsible for the 2003 epidemic, some of the key variables and their estimated values are listed in Box 2. Once these are measured, analyses of optimal disease mitigation interventions and their timings of introduction can be made.

Policy issues

Policy formulation for the control of an emerging pandemic is complex and will depend on many factors.

- The study of epidemic patterns and options for disease control needs to be conducted at regional, national, and international levels, since policy formulation and its implementation varied widely in recent pandemics. For both national and international policy makers, improving such surveillance should be an urgent priority.

- Assembling the world's leading scientists and medical researchers to provide a reliable information source for both national and international policy formulation is an urgent necessity. Governments often assemble national committees, irrespective of the expertise level within a country. A much better approach is to recognize that expertise from around the world should be integrated and used by all countries under the umbrella of an international agency — provided it chooses membership of an advisory committee on expertise and not international representation. Amongst the experts (e.g., influenza specialists in the case of an emerging influenza pandemic), it is essential to add generalists as well, since conventional wisdom in a narrow field can sometimes prove to be wrong! Broad expertise on advisory committees crossing infectious disease specialists, epidemiologists, clinicians, logistics experts, and communications specialists is essential.

- Alert levels must be based on case morbidity and mortality rates and decisions on what levels might require international alerts and actions.

- Policy makers need to ensure that the most modern tools, including mathematical models and simulation techniques, are used to guide recommended actions. These results then need to be modified in policy formulation by what is possible and what can be afforded.

- In recent epidemics and pandemics it has rarely (if ever) been clear what the main policy objectives are in national and international intervention efforts to mitigate disease. Policy objectives for mitigating infectious disease epidemics and pandemics should be transparently delineated. Some examples of possible policy objectives are listed in Box 3.
- Recent analyses suggest that some policy options for the control of epidemics conflict with other policy proposals. For example, it may not be possible to minimize the peak and duration of an epidemic with one set of interventions since "squashing" the peak tends to lengthen the duration of the epidemic (Hollingsworth et al., 2011). As such, policy makers need to be encouraged to list objectives in order of priority if all cannot be satisfied by the available intervention options, or if they conflict because of the dynamics of epidemic spread. The art of the possible is always a key issue in what can be done to mitigate impact as reflected in Box 4 for influenza A pandemics.
- Overall, the preceding recommendations highlight the key tasks for the policy makers: (i) establish the threat posed by the new infectious agent in terms of morbidity and mortality; (ii) assemble a panel of experts and "wise" generalists; (iii) identify what interventions are options and when they will be available; (iv) initiate simulating studies to see what works best and how much it will cost; (v) and, most importantly, define policy objectives clearly and in an order of priority.

References

World Health Organization (WHO). (2009). Pandemic influenza preparedness and response: A WHO guidance document. Retrieved Sept. 9, 2011, from http://whqlibdoc.who.int/publications/2009/9789241547680_eng.pdf

Hollingsworth, T. D., Klinkenberg, D., Heesterbeek, H., Anderson, R. M. (2011). Mitigation strategies for pandemic influenza A: Balancing conflicting policy objectives. PLoS Computational Biology, 7(2), 1–11

** A policy position paper prepared for presentation at the conference on Emerging and Persistent Infectious Diseases (EPID): Focus on Mitigation convened by the Institute on Science for Global Policy (ISGP) Oct. 23–26, 2011, at the University of Edinburgh, Edinburgh, Scotland.

Box 1: The emergence of a new infectious disease — urgent tasks

- Indication — unusual clusters of morbidity/mortality in space and time.
- Identify aetiological agent — demonstrate Koch's postulates.
- Develop a diagnostic test (serology and pathogen presence).
- Initiate research on drugs and vaccines — collaboration with pharmaceutical industry in diagnostics, treatment, and prevention.
- Activate data capture in real-time and communicate this information.
- Identify clinical algorithms for care of the sick.
- Identify and implement optimal public health measures for control.
- Keep public informed at all stages.

Box 2: Key variables for SARS

- Exposure to onset of symptoms (incubation period): mean 4.2 days.
- Onset of symptoms to admission to hospital — reflects rapidity of diagnosis: decreased from an average of 4.9 days at the beginning of the epidemic to less than 2 days by the mid-point of the epidemic. This variable affects the efficiency of isolation and quarantine in reducing transmission.
- Admission to hospital to death (for patients who died): mean of 23.5 days. This variable helps define the burden likely to fall on the health care system as the epidemic develops.
- Admission to hospital to discharge (for patients who recover): mean of 23.5 days.

Box 3: Policy objectives

- Minimize morbidity and mortality — with fixed or variable budget.
- Buy as much time as possible to wait for vaccine development.
- Minimize duration of the epidemic and impact on economy.
- Minimize peak prevalence below a defined level to avoid collapse of hospital care system.

Box 4: Intervention options for influenza A

- Any mitigation strategy requires very early detection and a well-planned plus rapidly executed response. Rapidity of the introduction of an intervention will depend on the resources made available to cover the entire duration of the epidemic.
- For rapidly spreading pathogens (respiratory or fecal/oral route of transmission) restricting entry of travelers from regions in which the pathogen is spreading is ineffective unless put in place early and it acts to restrict more than 99% of entries.
- Containment feasible to reduce peak incidence and the overall size of the epidemic using combinations of: prophylactic vaccines; antiviral agents to reduce morbidity/mortality and restrict the duration of infectiousness; increasing "social distance" by school/workplace/entertainment space closures, isolation, and travel restriction within a country.
- Simple public health measures such as the wearing of facial masks and hand-washing.
- Key questions for analysis by policy makers: Is any combination of the above capable of mitigating the epidemic and by how much? What interventions are available to me? How much do they cost? What are the resources available? What is the best combination? When do I introduce them and for how long?

Debate Summary

The following summary is based on notes recorded by the ISGP staff during the not-for-attribution debate of the policy position paper prepared by Prof. Sir Roy Anderson (see above). Prof. Sir Roy Anderson initiated the debate with a 5-minute statement of his views and then actively engaged the conference participants, including other authors, throughout the remainder of the 90-minute period. This Debate Summary represents the ISGP's best effort to accurately capture the comments offered and questions posed by all participants, as well as those responses made by Prof. Sir Roy Anderson. Given the not-for-attribution format of the debate, the views comprising this summary do not necessarily represent the views of Prof. Sir Roy Anderson, as evidenced by his policy position paper. Rather, it is, and should be read as, an overview of the areas of agreement and disagreement that emerged from all those participating in the critical debate.

Debate Conclusions

- Since the uptake of new technologies is often hindered by scientific, cultural, and bureaucratic barriers, the potential impact of these barriers must be considered, understood, and addressed to ensure the successful implementation of innovative technologies in disease mitigation.
- Disease pandemic policy objectives must be clearly developed and articulated for both policy makers and the public and the plans developed by governments to address pandemics need to be driven by, and thus aligned with, potentially distinct policy objectives.
- Effective communication of scientific information to politicians, other policy makers, and their staffs is a vital component of pandemic planning. Relationships with policy makers and their staffs must be built with trust over a longer time frame to be effective.
- While modelling is a pervasive and important tool in planning for pandemics, models must be based on assumptions that are transparent and consistent, and the limitations of any model and its outputs must be clearly explained and disclosed.

Current realities

Novel technologies for disease surveillance and monitoring, as well as new diagnostic and prognostic test methods to identify and characterize diseases, have been and continue to be developed. Such technologies were viewed as a rich resource for improving pandemic planning and response. Several examples of existing technologies that could be used to prevent or address an epidemic or pandemic were provided: saliva-based serology to ascertain infection and morbidity; data on air traffic passenger flow between major airports to predict the movement of epidemics; and mobile phone data to view individuals' movements and to determine who travels and/or spends significant time together. Specifically, it was opined that these technologies should have been employed to predict and mitigate the 2009 H1N1 influenza pandemic (PDM 2009 H1N1).

It was agreed that there are modern technologies that could help prevent and mitigate pandemics, but that epidemiology and public health have been slow to adopt these new tools. Some government organizations have recently begun to respond to this criticism. For example, the United Kingdom's Health Protection Agency (HPA) has recently heeded the criticism that it is lagging in the uptake of technology and has begun to address this problem.

While government planning for pandemic response and control was viewed as critical for protecting the public's health, there was consensus that current plans are generally suboptimal. For example, most countries published pandemic plans before PDM 2009 H1N1, but the specific policies and objectives in these plans were obscure. To illustrate this point, it was noted that it is challenging to discern from the published documents whether the policy objective is to control the pandemic or the epidemic. Furthermore, the definition of "control" is unclear in many existing plans (e.g., poor clarity on whether control means to minimize morbidity, mortality, the peak of an epidemic, or something else). Not only are the policy options often ambiguous, but it was also argued that they are frequently in conflict. One example was the effort to minimize both the peak and the duration of an epidemic, an effort which frequently represents contradictory goals. The logistics of pandemic response and control are also often poorly described. A specific example involved the review of one nation's PDM 2009 H1N1 plan by experts where the final plan provided by its creators inexplicably omitted much of the scientific rigor and scholarly input.

The importance of mathematical modeling as a critical tool in pandemic preparedness and planning was widely acknowledged. While those who are unfamiliar with models may be skeptical about the value of their applications to real problems, scientists commonly use models because they provide a method to quantify problems and to identify potential solutions that are not strictly based on qualitative opinions. While the mathematics that underpins modeling may often be considered the language of scientific communication, different mathematical methods can be used to create models (e.g., computer codes or equations). Additionally, the results from modeling can be communicated to policy makers and the public in a variety of ways (e.g., conceptually, verbally, or through diagrams, among other formats).

While the output generated through models may not provide the definitive "crystal ball" precision desired by policy makers, the media, and the general public, it was strongly argued that their quantitative foundation makes modeling a fundamental and essential part of disease pandemic preparedness. In particular, computational modeling is a useful technique to assist in scenario planning over a range of possibilities. This point was illustrated by the constructive results that emerged from recent models on the impact of closing schools over the course of an influenza pandemic. When modeled over a variety of scenarios (i.e., school closings at intervals of two, four, or six weeks after the inception of a pandemic), practical intervention information was elucidated regarding downgrading the importance of herd immunity and upgrading the influence of 5- to 10-year-old children in disease transmission.

It was noted that information provided to the public on infectious disease outbreaks often comes from news outlets (e.g., the BBC and CNN Web sites) rather than from governmental sources. For instance, most of the information the public received on PDM 2009 H1N1 came from the media — and the public rapidly absorbs information provided by the press. The 2002 to 2003 Severe Acute Respiratory Syndrome (SARS) epidemic was cited as an example of how the public more quickly reacted to recommendations provided by the media than to the government's pronouncement on what people should do to protect themselves.

Scientific opportunities and challenges

Several barriers that hinder the use of new technology for infectious disease prevention and mitigation were identified. For instance, the government agencies and organizations most involved in utilizing new technologies are currently under extreme fiscal pressure and, thus, are unable because of inadequate resources to implement new technology. Additionally, while a new method may represent a quantum leap from an informational and/or a cost-effectiveness perspective, it may still be difficult for a specific agency to commit incremental funding to such an implementation and conversion effort. Scaling up a technology from a laboratory environment to practical use or commercialization was also cited as a challenge because such efforts require significant time investments and unique skill sets. Organizations also may be less willing to embrace technologies that are externally developed. Since many government agencies have made significant financial and time investments in their data collection and management capabilities, each may be reluctant to adopt new technologies that render historical and newer data incompatible.

Privacy concerns related to the collection and sharing of health-related data, including ethical and security conflicts in making such data available to scientists, were viewed as a challenge to the development and use of simulations and modeling. In addition, the anonymization techniques used to ensure confidentiality are not always possible for small populations. The lack of publicly available data was also considered problematic. Mobile phone information, for example, is not accessible to the research community without agreements from mobile phone users.

While there was strong consensus that modeling is a useful tool for policy making and planning, there was also agreement that models should not be considered perfect. Modeling is a tool for the management of uncertainties, not a "crystal ball" that predicts with certitude. There will always be "unknowns" in models, which hinder their ability to accurately predict what will occur. Biological, sociological, and behavioral unknowns were highlighted as some of the areas where uncertainties can impact the predictive accuracy of models. For example, certain unknowns related to malaria affect the predictive abilities of models in terms of the acquisition of immunity. Since policy makers and the public inherently want absolute prediction and projection, the modeling community is often tempted to frame its findings in absolute terms. Effectively framing findings, including communicating unknowns, has long been a challenge for the modeling community. It was questioned to what extent the mathematical epidemiology community should move away from stating that its members can predict future outcomes and use that information to pick optimal policy options.

The Internet was described as an extraordinarily powerful tool that affords opportunities for gathering information about disease epidemics and pandemics which can potentially be used in epidemiological models. For example, there is current research that explores how well Web searches/hits on various Internet sites perform as an indicator of disease incidence. Web-based surveys were also considered a useful way to gather meaningful data. This was illustrated by a specific instance: during PDM 2009 H1N1, one country's health department set up a Web-based survey that collected weekly information from residents about their level of contact with other individuals (i.e., who and how often) and their influenza status.

This information was then mapped to provide snapshots of the pandemic's local progression.

The point was made that there is frequently a marked divergence between people's level of scientific knowledge and their behavior. For example, during PDM 2009 H1N1, U.K. physicians' vaccine uptake rate was exceedingly low. It was suggested that a Web-based interview approach would be useful for gathering information that could be used to disentangle the observed disconnect between knowledge and behavior.

Policy issues

In terms of policy formation, it was stressed that more precision is possible in defining and ranking policy objectives. It was strongly proposed that government planning must include detailed debates and internal discussions to expressly determine the order of priorities. To establish prioritized policies that are not in conflict with each other, scientifically credible advisers need to provide policy makers with a clear understanding of the published scientific literature as it pertains to formulating and analyzing policy options.

It was argued that it is imperative to introduce information on serology at the beginning of an epidemic to determine the prevalence of a disease in a population. Serological studies were not used at the outset of PDM 2009 H1N1, which led to the incorrect announcement that H1N1 was a serious pandemic. If serology had been initially conducted, analyses of test results would have demonstrated that PDM 2009 H1N1 was not as serious as originally predicted. It was asserted that the use of serology in the case of PDM 2009 H1N1 was slowed down by specialists who said they could not guarantee the specificity of the serological tests. However, it was noted that specificity is not important in emergencies of this kind. After the pandemic, WHO set up a small group to revise the criteria for declaring a disease as a pandemic. Hope was expressed that the WHO will use serology in its future guidelines for reclassifying an outbreak as a pandemic. The number of individuals infected in a population, as determined through serological studies, can be used to establish the nature of an infectious agent, specifically, whether a pathogen has: 1) high transmissibility, low pathogenicity; 2) low transmissibility, high pathogenicity; or 3) high transmissibility, high pathogenicity (the most dangerous).

Prior to developing an adequate serological test, agreement about the clinical definition of what is a "case" of the novel agent was deemed necessary. Agreement is difficult to come by, as evidenced by the different opinions and difficulty in developing a clinical case definition of SARS. Developing a clinical case definition requires improved information sharing by the clinical community about treatment profiles.

It was argued that because models can both influence policy and benefit public health, there is a need to use models more frequently in infectious disease-control efforts. To illustrate this point, a retrospective analysis of air traffic passenger flows between major world airports showed that these data could have been used to accurately predict the movement of PDM 2009 H1N1. Similarly, genomics (including whole genome sequencing) can be used to determine infectious disease transmission patterns. A caveat to using modeling for creating policy was that models may be specific to particular situations or countries, and therefore, universally applying findings may not be appropriate.

There was general agreement that scientists and physicians have a responsibility to effectively communicate complex science to policy makers, including the limitations associated with their studies and findings (e.g., models are tools to manage uncertainty and cannot be used to predict the future with absolute confidence). With respect to models, it was argued that poor communication frequently results in two scenarios — policy makers accept the model without question, which can cause future problems if they make decisions without fully understanding the model, or they hastily reject the model because their own incomprehension makes them wary. Compounding matters, in-person meetings between scientists and policy makers are frequently brief. Therefore, it was seen as vital that scientists be able to convey their messages both succinctly and clearly: communicating too much information is counterproductive, and simplicity in messaging is important. It was recommended that scientists predetermine the one single message they want to leave in the mind of a policy maker and focus on that area.

The effective use of information derived from scientific modeling for policy decisions requires the establishment of long-term, professionally respected relationships built on trust between the scientific community and those in government. The personalities of individuals in government were considered one of the most important factors to be considered in terms of influencing policy. Given the importance of interpersonal relationships, it was suggested that alternative paths of influence be considered if personality conflicts develop. Specifically, it was recommended that relationships be cultivated with those who influence policy makers, such as their staff and advisers. Additionally, military officials often have considerable influence and may be powerful allies. Frequent changeover within government positions is an area that complicates the process of developing relationships with the appropriate policy makers. It was therefore emphasized that new, valued relationships need to be continuously fostered.

The need to address privacy concerns and to be transparent in demonstrating how these concerns are managed was identified as important. Failing to properly address privacy concerns can often derail the ability to gather important monitoring information during an outbreak. For example, useful data can be collected in real time using technologies such as mobile telephones and social media. However, care needs to be taken initially, not only to randomize and anonymize the data, but also to be able to demonstrate clearly that privacy concerns have been considered throughout the collection and use of such data.

It was cautioned that models need to be based on assumptions that are transparent and consistent, and the strengths and limitations of any model and its outputs be clearly disclosed so that they can be inspected, criticized, and changed. To make policy makers more confident in the utility of models, an effort must be made to develop a "good practice" guide for modelers; this includes a Web site with explanations of the criteria that robust models need to follow. Additionally, the infectious disease community must look to other fields for guidance on how to gain the trust of policy makers in the results from models, particularly those fields that have been successful in influencing policy despite the inclusion of unknowns in mathematical computations (e.g., the climate change community).

In addition, a diversity of model predictions, based on different assumptions and unknowns, needs to be reviewed when employing model predictions for the creation of government policies; instead of relying on one model, the best three or four should be taken into consideration. Greater confidence in the findings from modeling can be generated when several agree on central points.

Flashy front-end packaging of models does not always signal that a model is scientifically or mathematically accurate. As such, it was emphasized that the "internal guts" (i.e., assumptions and calculations) of models be carefully reviewed by the scientific and medical communities before being presented to policy makers.

Multidepartmental government planning and response was highlighted as important. Strengths of different divisions vary and thus, could effectively be integrated. For example, logistical issues related to emergency management, such as managing the distribution of certain drugs (e.g., Tamiflu and Relenza to treat influenza), is a skill that the military has demonstrated successfully when it was asked to deal with drug distribution logistics during an outbreak. However, because interdepartmental collaboration can be challenging, it is often not done.

Proactive Use of Supply Chain Data in Foodborne Illness Outbreak Investigation**

Shaun Kennedy, B.S.Ch.E.
Director, National Center for Food Protection and Defense,
Assistant Professor, Veterinary Population Medicine,
University of Minnesota

Summary

Unfortunately, traditional epidemiological foodborne outbreak investigations are generally forensic. They allow us to know what went wrong so that preventive controls can be put in place for the future and we know where to assign blame for the outbreak. However, these investigations do not allow us to intervene and help those who will become ill because, with episodic contamination, the majority of the contaminated food is usually consumed before the epidemiologic investigation has identified the vehicle. Traditional epidemiological investigations are only really a mitigation strategy (i.e., interventional) for systemic contamination events in which there is low-level contamination over an extended period of time. Part of the challenge of the traditional epidemiologic approach is that we need outbreaks to be recognized before epidemiologists can carry out a case control study (i.e., identifying possible causal factors by comparing ill individuals to nonsick individuals). However, our primary detection system is currently the emergency room. When the investigation begins, the epidemiologist has to do extensive interviews to find out which foods to consider in the case control study. The more foods included, the longer the study takes — an inherent conflict. There is an opportunity to dramatically simplify these investigations by utilizing private sector supply chain data, but this requires strong public-private partnerships. In essence, by comparing the illness pattern with the specific product distribution patterns, one could identify which products are possible contamination vehicles. Using that data in a meaningful way, however, requires near real-time analysis of vast amounts of information. New approaches on how data from competitors could be combined without compromising proprietary business information or exposing companies to additional regulatory risk must be identified.

Current realities

Investigations of foodborne illness outbreaks that follow a "church picnic" scenario are relatively straightforward. If half of the picnic attendees ate the potato salad and the majority of them became ill, it is a fairly easy epidemiological investigation and the outbreak is over. However, this does not help those who became ill. Outbreaks such as the E. coli O104:H4 associated with sprouts in Germany, E. coli O157:H7 associated with spinach in the United States, Salmonella Saintpaul associated with peppers in the U.S., and many others, illustrate how the "church picnic" style investigation fails as a real mitigation strategy. In both E. coli cases, the epidemiological curve followed the basic trend as depicted in Figure 1; the consumption and illness presentation curves had already peaked before the vehicle was identified. In the case of Salmonella Saintpaul, some disease cases might have been prevented by the announcement to avoid peppers, yet it took months from the first illnesses to identify them as the vehicle. Thus, while the systemic nature of the contamination provided an opportunity to mitigate the consequences, the difficulty in identifying the source resulted in illnesses that could have been prevented by a more timely identification of peppers as the vehicle.

Supply chain data (i.e., information on how products move from pre-farm inputs, through primary production, harvest, and further processing, and to consumer purchase) were used in each case. However, the investigation and mitigation of the outbreak could have been accelerated if supply chain data had been more proactively and thoroughly utilized. As a normal part of the product traceback to try to identify the source, federal and local authorities obtained data on the products that they thought were most likely associated with the outbreak. However, real-time analysis of food supply chain data, as new illnesses become associated with an outbreak, was not and is currently not conducted. Real-time analysis would allow the list of foods and sources to be narrowed down, even before a clear association is identified or a traditional case control study is completed. The challenge is that the data would have to be collected and analyzed on a continual basis to be useful. For example, a single entity would have to receive data from all major retailers and mine these data as illnesses are identified.

In the Salmonella Saintpaul outbreak, initial inclusion of private sector data would have immediately indicated that the Florida tomatoes were likely not the source because the illness distribution exceeded the probable distribution of the Florida tomato harvest at that stage in the season. This investigation was the first time that import data available to U.S. federal agencies were significantly utilized prior to the identification of the probable vehicle, albeit in the final stages of the investigation, to narrow the number of possible sources from the more than 500 manufacturers and thousands of shipments during the outbreak. While in the Salmonella Saintpaul case investigators were looking at a limited segment of the food industry, for the U.S., there are more than 300,000 food producers who supply approximately 55,000 items for sale in roughly 900,000 retail outlets. Therefore, the brute force approach of manually reviewing each line entry would not be a realistic option.

Import data are the only type of real-time supply chain data currently available to federal officials. These data comprise only a small fraction of the existing supply chain data and are not usually shared with local officials or automatically analyzed to identify potential vehicles. Due to probable cost, it is not realistic for regulatory agencies to collect all available private sector data in real-time and on a continual basis. Also, companies are not likely to want their regulators to hold their proprietary data. Supply chain structure, for example, is part of how firms manage their cost structure. In some cases, businesses will not share company information on their suppliers with their customers, demonstrating how sensitive the food industry can be about basic supply chain structure.

Scientific opportunities and challenges

Import and supplier/customer data for each firm in the supply chain already exist, usually in electronic form. For most foods, however, these data are not held in one central database, even from supplier to retail outlet. Enterprise Resource Planning (ERP) systems or similar systems are widely deployed to manage, among other things, manufacturing systems, order fulfillment, and raw material/supplies acquisition. Import data are also available electronically. The scientific challenge is how to rapidly merge data from different sources, given that unfortunately there is no single, unifying information structure standard. The need to integrate disparate data is a challenge shared in many other contexts, from medical research to financial markets. As a result, the basic tools to analyze large, disparate datasets exist. The development of a system to acquire basic data on suppliers and production facilities of individual foods to retail outlets, down to the stock-keeping unit level, is therefore achievable. That alone would be a significant step forward as it would make it much easier to confirm that foods distributed in areas with no associated outbreak cases are not related to the specific outbreak. If the distribution pattern of a product matches some unique attribute of the illness distribution, it would conversely suggest that the product has a higher likelihood of being a source. In the Salmonella Saintpaul outbreak, there were higher incidences of illness in states where the implicated importer had distribution centers or more distribution than in other states. If that information had been available and/or considered during the investigation, produce items moving through those distribution centers could have been investigated as potential sources. Identifying this association becomes more difficult when the contaminated product is a widely used ingredient. It is at that point that trying to capture the sourcing data for the production facility, repacking house, or distribution center is important. Such investigations would drive a significant increase in data management complexity, but are still achievable. Imported ingredients dramatically increase complexity; while import data is available, there may be challenges with language barriers, limited electronic data capture/sharing capabilities, and compliance. If investigators want to trace all the way back to the farm, many products would be, at least for now, out of reach.

Policy issues

- The core technology exists to utilize supply chain data to accelerate outbreak investigations, and even at its simplest implementation, this would be a tremendous asset. There are a number of policy issues that must be addressed to ensure that supply chain data are effectively employed.
- It is necessary to accelerate outbreak investigation and source attribution without creating new regulatory enforcement or litigation hazards for the private sector. The requisite management and data needs of government agencies associated with the food system must also be defined.
- The reason for the food industry to share data in real-time must be justified, especially since there are associated costs (i.e., either direct and/or opportunity costs).
- The legal and regulatory framework for establishing an independent third party that can create a single unifying information structure and data standards — and should then become the clearinghouse for sharing supply chain data in the event of an outbreak — must be established.
- The private sector should fund a public supply chain surveillance system as part of the outbreak clearinghouse or as a separate entity, because it is the private sector that financially benefits from reducing the impact of unintentional food contamination and intentional food system events.
- A modest investment by the private sector to increase local public health capabilities for foodborne illness investigation would, according to the Council to Improve Foodborne Outbreak Response (CIFOR, 2009), significantly improve outbreak detection and response.

- The economic justification for the public sector enabling, and the private sector funding, these significant efforts is the reduction in losses to the public and the industry that would stem from accelerating outbreak source attribution. Beyond consumers, communities that would benefit economically from reducing consumer exposure in an outbreak include:
  - food businesses (especially retailers, finished food processors, and produce suppliers) who bear the direct cost of delayed or incorrect source identification
  - insurers of food businesses, as it reduces their overall exposure risk
  - health insurers, given that estimated U.S. direct health care related costs of foodborne illness are US$152 billion per year (Scharff, 2010)
- Developing the standards and protocols will not be easy, but the technology exists and the algorithms could be made. Only the will to collaborate in unconventional approaches to reduce the burden of foodborne illness is needed. The private sector investing in public infrastructure is a very different paradigm, but one that will protect the public and the private sectors. It is, however, somewhat of a misnomer to say that the private sector is paying, as in the end, it is always the consumer who pays.

References

Council to Improve Foodborne Outbreak Response (CIFOR). (2009). Guidelines for foodborne disease outbreak response. Retrieved September 19, 2011, from http://www.cifor.us/documents/CIFORGuidelinesFrontMatter_000.pdf

Scharff, R. L. (2010). Health-related costs from foodborne illness in the United States. Retrieved September 19, 2011, from http://www.producesafetyproject.org/media?id=0009

*** A policy position paper prepared for presentation at the conference on Emerging and Persistent Infectious Diseases (EPID): Focus on Mitigation convened by the Institute on Science for Global Policy (ISGP) Oct. 23–26, 2011, at the University of Edinburgh, Edinburgh, Scotland.*

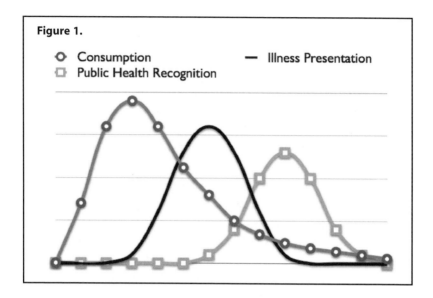

Figure 1.

O Consumption   — Illness Presentation
□ Public Health Recognition

Debate Summary

The following summary is based on notes recorded by the ISGP staff during the not-for-attribution debate of the policy position paper prepared by Prof. Shaun Kennedy (see above). Prof. Kennedy initiated the debate with a 5-minute statement of his views and then actively engaged the conference participants, including other authors, throughout the remainder of the 90-minute period. This Debate Summary represents the ISGP's best effort to accurately capture the comments offered and questions posed by all participants, as well as those responses made by Prof. Kennedy. Given the not-for-attribution format of the debate, the views comprising this summary do not necessarily represent the views of Prof. Kennedy, as evidenced by his policy position paper. Rather, it is, and should be read as, an overview of the areas of agreement and disagreement that emerged from all those participating in the critical debate.

Debate conclusions

- Foodborne diseases exert a heavy economic toll on the food industry, governments, and consumers. Better prevention and more rapid mitigation of outbreaks will reduce the overall expenditures required to manage food-related issues; therefore, proactive investments in food safety are needed.

- The complexity of the global food supply chain has substantially increased in recent years because of a steady rise in food imports/exports to and from countries around the world. Increasingly, regulatory agencies responsible for food safety do not understand the supply chain, leading to poor management and identification of outbreaks. Efforts must be made to be able to accurately trace the succession of food producers, suppliers, and retailers so measures can be implemented that reduce the prevalence and impact of foodborne disease outbreaks.

- Food safety standards, which require all global food sectors to follow the same basic safety criteria, must be implemented. Better harmonization of standards is increasingly important given the growing interconnectedness of the global food supply chain and the proliferation of multicomponent food products. However, as standards are raised, the ability of producers (particularly in less-wealthy countries) to finance increased safety costs and still compete in global markets must be taken into consideration.

- The incorporation of private-sector data into foodborne disease outbreak investigations is critical for improving the accuracy and speed with which the sources of outbreaks are identified. However, the food industry is unlikely to share its data directly with regulatory agencies because of economically motivated privacy concerns. It is therefore necessary for a third-party entity to act as a liaison between the private sector and regulatory agencies so that industry data can be utilized in an anonymous and harmonized manner that protects members' interests.

Partnerships between regulatory agencies and the food industry must also be expanded and encouraged. Both maintain separate, yet intertwined, roles in securing food safety. Since regulatory authorities have the capacity to set equitable standards and the food industry informs standards and influences compliance within supply chains, close cooperation is, and will continue to be, essential.

Current realities

There was general consensus that foodborne and waterborne diseases continue to be a major global issue that account for more than 2 billion cases of illness and 1 million fatalities each year worldwide. Incidents of foodborne diseases also carry a heavy economic burden related to decreased productivity and health care costs. In the United States alone, foodborne disease-related health care costs total approximately US$152 billion annually. Individual outbreaks also have significant economic costs, frequently forcing small businesses to close and larger ones to spend millions of dollars on product recalls. It was noted that (not including health care) most of the economic burden of foodborne diseases is borne by the private sector, wherein insurance companies and reinsurers shoulder much of the cost. The magnitude of these expenses was exemplified by a recent recall of peanut butter products, which was estimated to have cost the food industry between US$1 billion and US$1.5 billion.

The food supply chain has become increasingly globalized; countries, particularly in more-affluent regions, have been steadily expanding the amount of food products and ingredients that they source from other nations. This was underscored by the fact that the U.S. trades with all countries but one. It was recognized, however, that food safety is not globally consistent because efforts to address safety measures often compete against other issues, such as poor agricultural practices, minimum resources, and substandard public health infrastructure.

The identification and management of foodborne illness outbreaks were heavily discussed and it was concluded that both are currently inadequate, as exemplified by large outbreaks of foodborne diseases in the U.S. (e.g., *Salmonella* in peanut butter) and more recently in Germany (e.g., *E. coli* in sprouts). Several reasons for these identification and management shortcomings were identified, including the complexity of the food supply chain and the proliferation of multi-component foods/ingredients — both of which obscure the attribution of a pathogen to a particular food source. It was also contended that substandard public health infrastructures further complicate the identification and management of outbreaks because they are frequently linked to poor data availability and product recall obstacles. As a result, foodborne disease investigations have traditionally relied on emergency room reports to detect such outbreaks.

It was noted that, in some areas, proactive mechanisms to help facilitate traceback have been instituted. For example, the U.S. Food and Drug Administration (U.S. FDA) implemented a mandatory Reportable Food Registry (RFR), in which the food industry must report contamination issues discovered through its quality assurance programs. Once a problem is reported to the RFR database, the system calls for immediate "one step forward and one step back" traceback (i.e., to where a company sold its product and bought it from). While it was contended that the RFR database is a positive step toward proactively managing foodborne diseases, it was highlighted that the RFR only works in instances in which quality assurance has already detected a pathogen in food. Moreover, this form of traceback, while helpful, is insufficient because it does not work when the entire supply chain structure is not known. This is because one distributor may supply many wholesalers so even if a foodborne disease incident is mitigated by a retailer changing its wholesaler, other distributors may continue to buy the same product from a common supply source and perpetuate the problem by selling the product back to the original retailer.

It was generally agreed that the food industry considers much of the information it collects to be private data vital to members' business operations, providing market advantage, and a potential source of financial risk if not managed properly. As such, food companies infrequently share their data with regulatory authorities.

Attention was drawn to the role of retailers in food safety. Retailers have the ability to exert considerable pressure on food producers and processors to meet safety standards by refusing to sell products that do not meet their criteria. Such economic influence was considered a highly effective method for enforcing requirements that generally cannot be accomplished in the same way by regulatory authorities.

The discussion highlighted that the public does not have a firm understanding of the concept of risk related to food. While food supplies are often characterized simply as "safe" by regulatory authorities, this does not mean all food is, or can ever be, 100% safe. As such, it was contended that the public frequently takes safety proclamations at face value and does not discern that there are degrees of risk associated with food.

Scientific opportunities and challenges

The suggestion was made that the heavy economic burden of foodborne diseases could be offset by proactive investment in foodborne disease investigation systems. Simultaneously reducing food-related illnesses and associated expenditures could be attained by spending a fraction of the estimated US$152 billion that is currently spent on foodborne disease related health care.

There was skepticism over whether increasing usage of supply chain data by regulatory agencies and food inspectors could prevent foodborne disease outbreaks. Accordingly, it was recognized that better understanding of the supply chain will not prevent most *episodic* outbreaks. However, it was argued that having the ability to accurately trace foods and food products through the supply chain would create an opportunity to prevent *systemic* contamination at the grower and processor levels. This is considered particularly useful given that systemic outbreaks represent some of the largest outbreaks recorded in recent history. It was universally agreed that enhanced comprehension of the supply chain would facilitate more rapid and accurate identification of the source of an outbreak, which would thereby augment efforts to mitigate the spread of foodborne diseases.

The food industry's reluctance to share data with regulatory agencies was viewed as a significant challenge to large foodborne disease outbreak identification and subsequent mitigation because this information is a critical component of the supply chain needed to accurately and quickly identify the source of an outbreak. Moreover, incorporating private sector data into outbreak investigations, alongside data collected by regulatory agencies, would improve targeting of high-risk export countries or products so more rigorous sampling could be implemented where needed. While increased data sharing would improve food safety management, concerns were raised that small companies may not have the resources or infrastructure to share their information adequately. It was argued that large companies with good data management systems in place would be reluctant to participate in a system from which a portion of the industry was exempted.

A significant portion of the discussion focused on the effects of inconsistent food safety standards. Discrepancies in acceptable risk levels across areas where food is produced represent a critical challenge to ensuring that the global food supply is safe. While it was argued that standards should be harmonized to improve the performance of producers that currently employ substandard methods, it was simultaneously recognized that higher standards translate into higher production costs. Concerns were raised that higher standards and costs could hinder the ability of some producers to be economically competitive in the global market.

The point was raised that social, economic, and cultural systems are heavily intertwined. For example, changing people's behavior (e.g., related to hygiene) requires improvements in living standards. Adding to the complexity, the living standards of producers are tied to the market cost of the foods they sell. Efforts to improve living standards of individuals in low-income areas would necessitate increased production costs and the end-product prices of food on the global market. Paradoxically, end-product price increases would likely drive many of these producers out of business.

The development and implementation of technologies to improve food product traceback were discussed. Although the food industry has long been interested in using technology to enhance traceback mechanisms, progress has been slow. This obstacle was exemplified by the efforts of a large U.S. retailer to implement technologies that could improve the traceability of products within its supply chain. Despite more than a decade of radio frequency identification (RFID) technology investment, that retailer has been unable to achieve the goal of RFID tagging each consumer unit package due to its cost-prohibitive nature. Developing affordable technologies that can be applied to individual products therefore remains a challenge. However, it was noted that RFID tags have been successfully used at the pallet level and that increasing adoption of this technology for larger food lots could be an opportunity to improve product traceback. The use of RFID tags for animal tracking was also discussed. It was acknowledged that the use of RFID tags has had variable levels of success (e.g., animal tracking with RFID chips works fairly well in Europe, but not in the U.S.).

In terms of technologies for food safety, the use of irradiation to destroy harmful pathogens in food was highlighted as a process that is not used broadly enough. It was asserted that regulatory labeling requirements for irradiated foods hinder public acceptance. For example, in the U.S., labeling irradiated foods with the Radura symbol has not effectively conveyed to consumers that irradiated foods are safe and not radioactive. While expanding the amount of food that is irradiated was deemed a positive step toward improving food safety, it was acknowledged that the process does not work well for some foods (e.g., the shelf life is shortened for some produce and foods with a high fat content will not retain their original flavor unless they are irradiated frozen).

Data deficiencies were highlighted as an ongoing problem to ensuring food safety. It was noted that there is currently little data available on foodborne diseases in less-wealthy countries. Although the World Health Organization (WHO) has spent three years working on a project to estimate the global burden of foodborne illness, the project is expected to take another three years to complete due to poor food reporting systems in all world regions. Without better data, the full burden of foodborne illness cannot be understood.

Questions were raised as to whether hyper-vigilant food safety measures are creating microbe-naïve populations more susceptible to new diseases. It was argued that attempts to produce more sterile foods (i.e., foods free from pathogens) remove nonpathogenic microbes in the process. Many of these nonpathogenic microbes, such as those found in yogurt, are necessary for the human stomach to maintain a balanced number of flora. It was speculated that steep rises in the incidence of inflammatory bowel disease, ulcerative colitis, and Crohn's disease may be driven by efforts to remove pathogens from the food supply. A clear understanding of these linkages has yet to be established.

Policy issues

It was argued that regulatory agencies and foodborne disease investigators need access to the food industry's supply chain data to improve source attribution and outbreak identification. Moreover, it was underscored that proactive data sharing would be economically beneficial to the food industry. Broader usage of this information would minimize identification of the wrong source during an outbreak and thereby reduce the number of financially debilitating restrictions that are placed unfairly on incorrect food products. It was recommended that a third-party mechanism should be established to counterbalance the food industry's privacy concerns. By employing a third party to redact the data (so it does not include proprietary information or other confidential industry knowledge), private companies' willingness to share data would increase substantially. Although the ability of small food producers and processors to collect and disseminate data was questioned, it was argued that much of their supply chain information would be accounted for by larger processors and producers that typically buy from such smaller operations.

There was general agreement that food safety standards should be harmonized so that a minimum level of acceptability is achieved worldwide. Because the costs associated with safety criteria frequently dissuade producers from following safety guidelines, it was argued that regulatory agencies should set universally mandatory performance standards to reduce the likelihood of economically motivated noncompliance caused by market competition. Higher standards will increase production costs, and therefore raise the end-product cost to the consumer. However, it was asserted that there is already a cost to the consumer related to foodborne illness, regardless of the approach. Furthermore, proactively improving safety at the production level is more cost-effective than reactively controlling foodborne outbreaks. In terms of enforcement, it was argued that the food industry, particularly retailers, must take the lead in ensuring that minimum standards are upheld.

Increasing research into foodborne disease transmission was highly recommended. To prevent and mitigate these diseases in humans, a greater understanding of the pathogens involved in foodborne diseases is required. Likewise, investment should be made in developing rapid diagnostic tools, which are also affordable to low-income areas, so that outbreaks can be more broadly prevented.

Underinvestment in public health infrastructures among all world sectors was highlighted as a significant challenge to the identification of food safety. It was noted that infrastructural deficiencies in less-wealthy countries are caused by too few funds spread across competing priorities. Similarly, public health infrastructure investments have declined in more-wealthy countries due to the presently weak economic climate globally. It was argued that increasing investments in public health infrastructures is required to improve outbreak identification, expand source attribution, and reduce overall public health losses. This was considered particularly important given the global nature of the food supply.

Because both the public and private sectors maintain integral roles in ensuring food safety, it was asserted that public-private partnerships should be encouraged and developed. Including the private sector in public research activities was considered one step toward achieving this goal. It was further proposed that by facilitating greater information-sharing and common goals, such relationships would be mutually beneficial. Moreover, strong sentiments were expressed that food safety policies will be most effective if these two groups work together because they retain interdependent functions. For example, authoritative bodies are needed to set far-reaching standards that take into consideration the needs of all groups along the supply chain, while at the same time industry is needed to inform setting of standards, collect supply chain data, and stimulate economic incentives for compliance.

Opportunities for Mitigating Foodborne Illnesses Caused by Emerging and Persistent Infectious Agents**

Michael P. Doyle, B.Sc., M.Sc., Ph.D.
Regents Professor and Director, Center for Food Safety,
University of Georgia

Summary

Foodborne illnesses caused by infectious agents are a major, global public health concern (e.g., a recent outbreak of E. coli O104 infection caused more than 50 deaths). The international food trade has grown exponentially during the past decade, especially from developing countries where sanitary practices are often subpar and foodborne pathogen contamination is prevalent. In many countries, antibiotics critical to human therapy are used indiscriminately in food production, resulting in the development of multiple antibiotic resistance in foodborne pathogens. In addition, many developing countries are the principal global providers of sensitive ingredients that are sources of harmful microbes. Two critical needs to enhance the safety of the global food supply are the development of: 1) rapid methods to sample foods and detect foodborne pathogens and 2) effective treatments to kill harmful microbes while retaining the fresh-like characteristics of raw foods. Opportunities for international policies to greatly influence the mitigation of foodborne disease outbreaks include: (i) widely implementing a global surveillance and outbreak investigation system, (ii) requiring the development and implementation, by the food industry, of comprehensive food safety plans, (iii) developing and implementing robust sampling procedures and rapid methods for detecting pathogens in sensitive food ingredients and ready-to-eat foods, and (iv) globally restricting the use of antibiotics, which are important to human therapy, in agricultural production.

Current realities

Current estimates indicate that almost 50 million cases of foodborne illness occur annually in the United States, of which the infectious agents norovirus, Salmonella, Campylobacter, Shiga toxin-producing E. coli, and Shigella are the principal known causes. Produce, followed by fish, poultry, meat, and shellfish, are the leading vehicles of recent foodborne outbreaks. Fresh fruits and vegetables have become major vehicles of foodborne illnesses in the United States and Europe. About one-fourth of foodborne outbreaks reported in the U.S. in 2006 were associated with produce, and most were from leafy greens that were fresh-cut, bagged, and ready-to-eat.

Recent advances in the Centers for Disease Control and Prevention's (CDC) and U.S. state health departments' surveillance and outbreak investigation systems have led to the identification of many new vehicles of foodborne outbreaks, including bagged spinach, peanut butter, ground pepper, and jalapeno peppers. These systems have been important in identifying: (i) new foodborne pathogens, (ii) new risky food processing and distribution practices, (iii) foods or ingredients not previously recognized as high-risk, and (iv) "problem" suppliers and food processors, both domestic and international (Tauxe et al., 2010). Sensitive ingredients that are added to ready-to-consume foods that generally do not receive an additional microbial kill treatment are a major public health concern in the food safety net. Foods that contain these sensitive ingredients include ice cream, nutrition bars, cooked or fermented meat products, and snack foods. Types of sensitive ingredients include peanut and nut butter/paste, chocolate, nuts, spices, herbs, flour, and vitamins. Salmonella contamination is the principal concern associated with sensitive ingredients; it can produce serious illness in people even when present in small numbers — less than 1 Salmonella organism/gram.

Most developed countries are importing foods at unprecedented rates, largely from developing countries such as China, India, Mexico, and Brazil (Doyle, 2009). Currently, about 20% of the U.S. food supply, and many sensitive ingredients, including about 45% of tree nuts and most spices, is imported. Sanitation practices for food production and processing are not universally equivalent throughout the world, and major weaknesses occur in many developing countries. Spices, nuts, produce, and seafood are examples of food items in which Salmonella contamination has resulted from poor sanitary practices (Doyle and Erickson, 2008).

In addition, antibiotics, including those critical for human therapy, are extensively applied indiscriminately and inappropriately in some developing countries to prevent and control contamination of harmful microbes in livestock, poultry, and aquaculture. China has the world's most rapid growth rate of antimicrobial resistance: Resistance rose approximately 22% between 1994 and 2000. A recent study of antimicrobial resistance of Salmonella isolates from chickens in China revealed that more than 85% of Salmonella Indiana (a dominant serotype) isolates were highly resistant to 10 antibiotics, and many of these isolates were resistant to 16 antibiotics. A large proportion of these antibiotics, which the microbes are resistant to, are critical for human therapy.

Scientific opportunities and challenges

One of the greatest impediments to verifying the safety of foods is the lack of rapid (real-time) methods that would enable sampling large volumes of foods and testing them for hazardous contaminants, such as infectious agents. Pathogen tests, including molecular-based methods, typically take many hours (e.g., 24 hours) to complete, and the sample size is relatively small (e.g., 25 grams or a total of 375 grams from 60 samples). These methods are not conducive to determining the safety of large shipments of food. Reliable, sufficiently sensitive, rapid pathogen-detection methods, which preferably take less than one hour, are needed to enable more rapid test and release programs. In addition, advanced methods are needed to concentrate samples, thereby enabling testing of large volumes of foods for more meaningful results.

Fresh produce has become recognized as a leading vehicle of foodborne disease outbreaks, in part because of the lack of available, cost-effective treatments (other than cooking or irradiation) that can both kill pathogens and retain the desired fresh-like characteristics of fruits and vegetables. Fresh-cut produce (e.g., lettuce, celery) is especially difficult to disinfect because most treatments degrade the quality of cut fruits and vegetables (e.g., browning, wilting), and harmful microbes can become internalized in the cut tissue where chemical treatments cannot contact them. Hence, there is a pressing need for the development of highly effective antimicrobial treatments that retain the quality of fresh and fresh-cut fruits and vegetables (e.g., sprouts).

Policy issues

- The best overall mitigation strategy for global reduction of emerging and persistent foodborne infectious disease outbreaks is to require the food industry to develop and implement food safety plans based upon approved models. These plans should include good agricultural practices for food producers, as well as hazard analysis and pathogen control points for food processors. The Food and Agricultural Organization (FAO) should be responsible for developing the model food safety plans and assisting the food industry with their implementation, especially in the developing world. The Codex Alimentarius should be responsible for establishing not only guidelines, but also global requirements for the application of food safety plans by the international food industry.

- A more widely implemented global surveillance and outbreak investigation system for human foodborne illnesses, which includes better food source attribution and traceback than currently exists, is needed to mitigate outbreaks of foodborne illness. Not all food producers and food processors are equally committed to producing safe foods given that their primary driver is generally economics/low cost. Such a system should be managed globally by the World Health Organization (WHO) and FAO working in conjunction with country health and agriculture departments. This would enable detection of otherwise unrecognized outbreaks, better identification of the vehicle (food) transmitting the outbreak strain, and more rapid implementation of control measures to minimize the number of illnesses globally.

- Development and implementation of robust sampling and rapid methods for detection of foodborne pathogens in sensitive ingredients could mitigate the risk of foodborne outbreaks. Globally, FAO should provide oversight of the development of sampling and rapid detection procedures and Codex should globally implement their usage.

- Ready-to-eat foods that do not receive an additional pathogen kill step following the addition of sensitive ingredient(s) (e.g., spices, chocolate, nuts, nut paste), as well as ready-to-eat foods considered to be of high risk to humans (e.g., sprout seeds and fresh-cut fruits/vegetables) found to be contaminated in international trade, should be reported to a global electronic portal developed and maintained by FAO or a reputable private entity.

- The use of antibiotics that are important for human therapy in agricultural production should be restricted to application by veterinarians and not made available directly to food producers. Prescribing practices among veterinarians could be improved by following electronic medical guidelines for the use of specific antibiotics, or antibiotic alternatives, for treating or preventing animal diseases. FAO and WHO should be responsible for developing prudent antibiotic use criteria and Codex should implement the rules for restricted antibiotic application by veterinarians.

References

Doyle, M.P. (2009). From wild pigs and spinach to tilapia and Asia: The challenges of the food safety community. (The John H. Silliker Lecture). Food Protection Trends, 28:800–03.

Doyle, M.P., & Erickson, M.C. (Eds.). (2008). Food imports: Microbiological issues and challenges. Washington DC: ASM Press.

Tauxe, R.V., Doyle, M.P., Kuchenmüller, Schlundt, J., & Stein, C.E. (2010). Evolving public health approaches to the global challenge of foodborne infections. International Journal of Food Microbiology, 139(Suppl. 1):S16–28.

*** A policy position paper prepared for presentation at the conference on Emerging and Persistent Infectious Diseases (EPID): Focus on Mitigation convened by the Institute on Science for Global Policy (ISGP) Oct. 23–26, 2011, at the University of Edinburgh, Edinburgh, Scotland.*

Debate Summary

The following summary is based on notes recorded by the ISGP staff during the not-for-attribution debate of the policy position paper prepared by Dr. Michael Doyle (see above). Dr. Doyle initiated the debate with a 5-minute statement of his views and then actively engaged the conference participants, including other authors, throughout the remainder of the 90-minute period. This Debate Summary represents the ISGP's best effort to accurately capture the comments offered and questions posed by all participants, as well as those responses made by Dr. Doyle. Given the not-for-attribution format of the debate, the views comprising this summary do not necessarily represent the views of Dr. Doyle, as evidenced by his policy position paper. Rather, it is, and should be read as, an overview of the areas of agreement and disagreement that emerged from all those participating in the critical debate.

Debate conclusions

- As a significant cause of morbidity and mortality worldwide, foodborne diseases must be effectively controlled to protect human health and to limit health care costs in all countries. While less-affluent countries bear a disproportionate burden from foodborne diseases in terms of both illness and death rates, wealthier countries experience high levels of food-related morbidity and significant health care-related expenditures.

- The continuing demand for cheaper food products in more-affluent countries discourages food-exporting nations from establishing and regulating rigorous food safety systems since such costs often offset much of the initial savings associated with producing food inexpensively in less-affluent countries. Thus, the financial pressures found in the competitive global markets discourage exporters from implementing the safer agricultural and monitoring practices designed to prevent foodborne diseases.

- Since the early identification of pathogens in food is limited by currently available testing methods, it is critical that significant improvements be made in the real-time diagnostic tests and sampling methodologies if the impact of foodborne diseases on humans is to be mitigated. Regulatory agencies (e.g., the United States Food and Drug Administration [U.S. FDA]) do not currently have the technical or logistical capacity to test the number of food samples required for timely and comprehensive pathogen detection.

- Both the incorrect and excessive use of antibiotics in food production are increasingly important issues that require veterinarians and producers to stringently control the proper use of antibiotics in animals within the food chain. Regulatory agencies must ensure that the practices used in administering antibiotics accurately identify those problematic food products that must be rapidly banned from importation to protect human health.

- Improved educational programs that focus on stakeholders at every level of the food supply chain, including food suppliers, the public, and the press, must be established to identify the appropriate measures to be followed in preventing foodborne disease outbreaks and to mitigate the spread of these diseases once an outbreak has been identified.

Current realities

It was acknowledged that foodborne diseases are a significant problem worldwide. Less-wealthy countries were highlighted as bearing most of the mortality burden associated with foodborne diseases. However, it was stressed that although morbidity (i.e., food-related illness) is also more prevalent in less-wealthy areas, it is, nevertheless, a serious issue in all global sectors. This was exemplified by the 2011 outbreak of Shiga toxin-producing *Escherichia coli* (*E. coli*) in Germany where there were approximately 50 deaths, 900 cases of haemolytic uremic syndrome (a complication of an infection that can lead to kidney failure), and thousands of cases of diarrhea. In terms of demographic breakdowns, infants, young children, the elderly, and immunocompromised individuals were pinpointed as the groups most susceptible to foodborne disease. However, those in other age brackets who are healthy can also be at risk.

A recent survey by the Pew Charitable Trusts has shown that after economic issues, food safety is the primary concern of the public in the U.S. The effectiveness of lobbying by consumers in affluent countries such as the U.S. for strong policies to ensure food safety has been routinely demonstrated. For example, U.S. parents who have lost children to infectious disease outbreaks associated with food were highly effective in lobbying legislatures for better food safety policies even though the total mortality rates were low.

There was general agreement that in addition to being a major public health concern, foodborne diseases are often critical economic issues as well. This was exemplified by the economic impact of foodborne illness in the U.S., which annually costs the nation US$152 billion in health care. Such high expenditures were perceived to be largely due to costs associated with the treatment of morbidity, particularly for the elderly whose health care is largely paid by the social insurance program Medicare.

The debate also highlighted the increasingly global nature of the food supply, as exemplified by the changing origins of food consumed in the U.S. For example, 50% of the fruits and vegetables consumed in the U.S. are now imported from Southeast Asia. Seafood is also imported in similarly high proportions from Asian countries, including China.

Economic issues were underscored as driving forces in the globalization of the food supply. As an example, current manufacturing practices were contrasted with past food supply-chain models — in the U.S., food was previously produced locally and then shipped overseas for repackaging before being reimported. Today, these same products are frequently both grown and packaged outside the U.S. This shift is largely due to lower labor costs in less-wealthy countries, since labor accounts for approximately 40% of the cost of production. It was argued that within 20 years more than half of the food consumed in the U.S. will be imported from less-affluent countries, many of which may have production standards and public health infrastructure that are inferior to those generally found to be acceptable in the U.S.

It was recognized that issues related to food production are politically charged and that countries have different ethical and regulatory standards, which can result in societal challenges to the implementation of scientifically credible and effective food safety practices. Examples of products that were intentionally contaminated to increase profits (i.e., economically motivated adulteration) include melamine in milk, chloramphenicol in honey, and antibiotics in vitamins. In these instances, it was noted that proper regulatory standards are either nonexistent or disregarded.

There was general consensus that antibiotic resistance is an ongoing and growing obstacle to ensuring food safety, particularly in foods originating from less-wealthy countries and/or countries where there is poor oversight of food production. In these cases, antibiotics are often used in place of good agricultural practices (GAP) or to correct the consequences of poor agricultural practices. China is an example of a country where antibiotic resistance is of particular concern. Antibiotic-resistant pathogens are routinely transported across borders with the movement of food products and ingredients.

It was acknowledged that, given the amount of imported food products, regulatory agencies even in more-wealthy countries are often unable to manage the volume of testing required to ensure food safety.. Given the recognition that representative proportions of food products are not adequately inspected or tested, it was acknowledged that better real-time tests and more effective sampling protocols are urgently needed. The U.S. FDA was identified as one of the regulatory agencies severely hampered in fulfilling its mandate due to a lack of capacity and resources. Of the goods imported into the U.S., less than 1% are visually inspected or sampled.

It was repeatedly mentioned that there are many tiers of food safety acceptability, as well as differing rules, guidelines, and regulations, within and between countries. Regulatory agencies sometimes set policies that are difficult, if not impossible, to implement. Such policies include zero tolerance for particular pathogens in food (e.g., salmonella in poultry) or banning food preservatives, such as sorbate, without providing viable alternatives.

Part of the discussion focused on the current role of the food industry in food safety. It was clear that while some producers do engage in poor or illicit practices (e.g., adulterated food), this is not a general problem. From an economic perspective, much of the food industry has a strong self-interest in ensuring that food is safe because of the economic repercussions of foodborne disease outbreaks or the sale of hazardous food (i.e., the inability to export, negative consumer reactions/lobbying).

The U.S. food industry has been strongly supportive of food safety. This was exemplified by its support of the recent FDA Food Safety Modernization Act (including lobbying Congress to pass the bill) and lobbying for more funding for the FDA. While it was argued that the changes included in the FDA Food Safety Modernization Act were not as extensive as were needed, it was generally agreed that the modifications were a positive step.

Retailers were identified as having a greater impact on decisions throughout the entire food chain, including the producer level, than regulatory agencies. This impact extends to what products are sold based on consumer demand (e.g., reluctance to sell genetically modified foods based on consumer opinion).

Scientific opportunities and challenges

The existence of extremely large and cumbersome regulatory systems that have not adapted to the regulatory requirements based on 21st century scientific understanding, and thus are often counterproductive, was considered a major challenge to the effective implementation of food safety standards. These regulatory systems are not only unwieldy due to their size and complexity, but they are also territorial. Improvements were viewed as directly connected to increased dialogues between scientists who work with new technologies and policy makers who need to better understand how these technologies can improve the regulation of food safety.

It was also recognized that a significant challenge to food safety management is the inability of regulatory agencies to adequately inspect imported products. The large volume of imports into more-affluent countries prohibits the visual inspection of each product. Instead, inspection is managed through a system of sampling. Yet it was understood that such sampling protocols are inadequate. Sampling large batches of a food product remains a challenge that has not been solved. Rapid diagnostic testing and improved sampling methodologies would increase the capacity of regulatory agencies to more quickly identify a problem with a particular food or ingredient. Efforts to improve food inspection through technological advancements are under way, including a new generation of microbiological testing that could pave the way for shorter and more effective pathogen detection.

The complex nature of the food supply chain has given rise to a number of products being characterized as stealth foods or ingredients (i.e., ingredients such as spices that are frequently incorporated into other food products and therefore become difficult to identify as the source of an outbreak). It is difficult to identify stealth foods or ingredients as a source of contamination because of their ubiquitous use in numerous products.

The complexity of the food supply chain has been increased by the introduction of pathogens in food that may be present in a viable, but nonculturable form. Current techniques, though able to identify genetic material of these pathogens, may not be able to discriminate between live and dead organisms, nor are they able to do so in real time. New, more versatile techniques and detection tools are needed to address this challenge, including increasing proactive real-time detection of pathogens in food products before they cause illness in the consumer.

There was consensus that efforts undertaken by the food industry and regulatory agencies to educate the public, suppliers, and media on matters related to food safety and foodborne diseases are currently inadequate. While programs to educate consumers do exist, foodborne disease outbreaks that could have been prevented had consumers followed the recommended instructions indicate that the public is either not receiving sufficient information or not accepting the advice provided. Likewise, producers still frequently engage in poor food safety practices, demonstrating an inadequate level of educational outreach. It was also made clear that the media requires better education on how to correctly convey food safety information to the public.

The importance of understanding social and cultural factors affecting the burden of foodborne diseases was underscored. For example, in Japan, even though the population is highly conscious of food safety, cultural norms of eating raw fish and meats persist. While the government implemented strict food safety laws for industry to control this practice, there is potential for resistance from the public against such regulations. Nonetheless, such information provides consumers with an opportunity to alter their attitudes and thereby empowers governments to pressure the food industry to make changes.

While socioeconomic factors were recognized as playing an important role in the production and consumption of safe food, more research concerning these factors is needed to provide a better perspective on how to create balanced policies that enlist public participation in reducing foodborne disease burdens.

Many farmers often may not understand the implications and consequences of properly using antibiotics in food production. Educational programs to inform farmers about the problem of creating antibiotic resistance and GAP were considered necessary to improve food safety at the production stage in the food supply chain.

Obtaining a practical balance between the costs associated with food safety and food pricing in global markets was considered a focal point for finding an appropriate approach to setting reasonable food safety standards worldwide. While additional expenses will be incurred by food producers in lower-income areas to meet constantly changing safety standards, the resultant food products are likely to become more acceptable in those markets that demand higher food safety. Simultaneously, the costs associated with food safety will cause the production costs in less-wealthy and wealthy countries to become similar, thereby reducing the financial advantages of production previously found in less-wealthy countries.

Cheaper sources of food were commonly thought to involve the sacrifice of some elements of food safety, often leading to foodborne disease problems that negate any initial economic benefits.

Policy issues

Extensive dialogue focused on the cost/benefits of making changes to current foodborne disease management systems. It was argued that, in wealthier countries, there has been great success in reducing the number of deaths related to foodborne diseases and that increased expenditure would therefore not reduce mortality enough to warrant the costs. The counterpoint was made that although mortality associated with foodborne disease has been dramatically reduced, the considerable morbidity experienced by wealthier countries has a significant impact on the health, productivity, and fiscal expenditures of these regions. Because of the high costs associated with treating foodborne illnesses, mitigating foodborne disease outbreaks is generally a more cost-effective route than reacting to the problem after the fact.

It was suggested that the Food and Agriculture Organization (FAO) be responsible for developing quality assurance measures along the food supply chain and improving food safety on a global scale. In terms of quality assurance, these FAO efforts need to be directed at imported food and food ingredients from less-wealthy countries. The suggestion was strongly contested, however, by those who felt that this task fell outside the FAO's mandate as an organization that is largely concerned with poverty reduction. It was argued that the food industry may be more effective than an international organization at ensuring the compliance of producers along the food chain. Alternatively, the more-affluent countries, together with food production companies, could take overall responsibility for food safety in which a bottom-up approach, through government oversight integrated with country-to-country agreements, would promote food safety at the grassroots level.

Questions were raised as to who is responsible for setting safety standards. Some advocated on behalf of international organizations; others proposed that standards reflect the needs of individual countries. Those in favor of an international model argued that cohesive standards would give producing countries (particularly in less-affluent regions) a greater voice in dictating what can be done to protect food at realistic world-market prices. When producers are not part of the conversations used to set food safety standards, standards are frequently determined by importing countries, but are not met in general. Those in favor of a country-to-country model argued that international standards assume that all importing countries have the same food safety ideals, when in reality this is not the case (e.g., some countries will accept genetically modified foods and others will not). Such disagreements often result in food safety standards becoming major international trade issues.

It was recommended that public-private partnerships need to be established that make use of the tremendous impact private companies have on their own food supply chains. These companies are able to foster change at any point along the supply chain through the economic incentives that reward the purchase of specific products. Collaboration between regulatory agencies and the private sector to develop food safety standards and enforcement regulations is required to establish a higher level of implementation of the rules and better compliance by producers and suppliers. However, caution was expressed as to how much new regulation is placed on the food industry, as it already contends with significant layers of policies.

Political and economic forces were considered essential in the development of food safety measures, as well as in broader conceptualizations of what constitutes safe food. For example, global markets, where food is exchanged between areas of differing political, economic, and geographic backgrounds, demonstrate the disadvantages associated with the distribution of unsafe food among different regions of a given country, even when food safety standards are in place. Establishing food safety rules and regulations that satisfy all stakeholders was seen as an essential step in effective regulation.

It was noted that the Codex Alimentarius, created jointly by FAO and the World Health Organization (WHO), is a highly politicized organization in which certain countries drive the agenda. Despite the benefits of Codex as a global reference point on food codes, political impediments make Codex not as effective as it could be in addressing food safety. The question was raised as to how Codex might be depoliticized, but it was acknowledged that there is no clear way to achieve this.

Several suggestions were raised as ways to move forward in combating the economically motivated adulteration of food products and ingredients. First, because some countries do not place enough importance on preventing adulteration, multinational companies buying food products need to place direct pressure on producers to comply with food safety standards. Second, to protect consumers from contaminated products, banning products from particular countries must be used as a prevention measure. However, the potential trade implications of such actions must be considered. Third, efforts are needed to encourage a culture change, wherein the producers would be educated and encouraged to view adulteration as an unacceptable practice.

Interest was expressed in promoting food safety through trade agreements and in exploring what impact this would have on World Trade Organization (WTO) agreements. It was contended that because large quantities of food are imported and exported, any implemented food safety regulations that affect food products would become a trade issue. It was suggested that attempts should be made to embed matters of public good related to food safety into trade treaties dealing with food.

It also was suggested that increased educational programs on foodborne diseases are necessary, and would have a greater impact on public understanding and acceptance of regulations. The material of these educational programs must be tailored to reach the desired audiences, which differ by socioeconomic status, culture, and nationality, among other classifications.

There was consensus on the need to change the culture of the food industry that comprises the global food supply chain, but opinions differed on how best to accomplish such a change. Some advocated on behalf of implementing GAP, educating industry stakeholders (e.g., providing technical training and teaching why certain practices are necessary), and globally harmonizing standards. These proposals were countered by those in favor of a culture change within the regulatory agencies to make better use of available resources and to better understand the implications and nuances of a global food supply chain. Still others suggested that private food companies would be best positioned to elicit cultural changes along the supply chain by working at the local level to ensure standards are met.

Three potential avenues for limiting antibiotics in food products were presented: 1. Veterinarians need to be given full oversight over antibiotic applications to mitigate against improper use; 2. Producers (particularly on small farms) need to be informed about the critical importance of the best practices associated with antibiotics and the need for proper supervision; 3. Certain products (e.g., honey tainted with the antibiotic chloramphenicol) must be banned from importation. While these actions are important, they can lead to trade issues with the WTO.

Although foodborne diseases impact all world sectors, it was argued that the disparity in the disease burden between more- and less-affluent areas must be addressed. Cost-effective efforts to prevent poor food safety practices in low-income countries (e.g., antibiotics in milk) must be implemented. It may be helpful for international agencies such as WHO to become involved because of the strong links between deficient food safety practices and poverty.

The issue of food security (i.e., the adequate availability of healthy food for human consumption) was also raised during the discussion. There was consensus that, primarily in less-wealthy countries, food security may be more of a concern than food safety. This means that countries may opt to direct limited resources toward providing an affordable and nutritious food supply for its population.

Synthetic Biology: A New Weapon in Our War Against Infectious Diseases**

John I. Glass, Ph.D.
Professor, J. Craig Venter Institute

Summary

Prior to the modern age, infectious diseases were the principal cause of human morbidity and mortality. The invention and widespread use of vaccines and antibiotics, along with advances in public health, sanitation, and nutrition, expanded human lifespan. Nevertheless, a variety of recent changes in society has increased the infectious disease burden globally. Although the discovery of new antibiotics has become more difficult, and the cost and time to licensure of new vaccines has increased, advances in biology offer possibilities for mitigating infectious diseases. Synthetic biology is a new field that engages in the design and assembly of genes and chromosomes from chemically synthesized DNA to create cells with properties unobtainable by conventional methods. It is already providing new ways to produce antibiotics and vaccines. Future advances in methods for DNA synthesis will make experimentation using synthetic bacteria and viruses less expensive and faster. This technology will enable the creation of vaccines based on rationally designed bacteria and viruses. Unfortunately, this technology could also enable bioterrorism. Recent construction of a bacterial cell with a synthetic genome showed that it currently would be too difficult for bioterrorists to synthesize bacterial pathogens; however, the use of synthetic biology to construct viruses is vastly easier. Still, the potential benefits of synthetic biology far outweigh the risks.

Current realities

In 1967, United States Surgeon General William Stewart wrote to Congress, "It is time to close the book on infectious diseases." If only that statement were true. It was made at a time when antibiotic drug discovery and vaccine development were in their heyday. Advances in public health such as nutrition, insect control, and water and sewage treatment all made the elimination of infectious diseases seem possible. In hindsight, such optimism seems naive.

Today our view of infectious diseases is quite different. We have new and emerging disease agents, such as HIV. Although existing drugs still work in most cases, pathogens have evolved resistance mechanisms for all current antibiotics. Old scourges like tuberculosis (TB) have emerged in multidrug-resistant forms that defy all treatment. New phenomena, such as an aging population, increasing numbers of immunocompromised patients, and rapid international travel increase vulnerability to infectious disease. New antibiotic development, which peaked in the 1980s, has slowed greatly. Many pharmaceutical companies have abandoned infectious disease research because of a failure to find new antibiotics in their chemical libraries, and the realization that development of resistance to new antibiotics would render them ineffective prior to patent expiration. Vaccines are now also becoming less effective because of another kind of resistance: the myth that all vaccines are dangerous. This distrust of vaccines has resulted in the avoidance of immunization and increased susceptibility to pathogens previously under control, which has triggered new epidemics.

Nonetheless, even though the war against infectious diseases may never be won, scientific advances continue to enable development of new weapons to combat pathogens. Genomics (i.e., reading and understanding DNA sequences) and synthetic biology are fields that provide insight into how an organism functions by reading its genetic code and enabling large-scale genetic remodeling via synthesis of genes and genomes. Biological experimentation provides insight needed to build new organisms and viruses that can be used to solve human problems.

The J. Craig Venter Institute (JCVI) Synthetic Biology Group is using synthetic biology to accelerate and improve the manufacture of influenza virus vaccines. One of the greatest threats to public health would be the emergence of a new pandemic strain of influenza virus that could claim millions of lives before a vaccine can be made. Because the virus is constantly evolving, every influenza season requires a new vaccine to be designed and produced based on the most important circulating viral strains. Every year, vaccine makers begin a six-month race to produce hundreds of millions of doses of vaccine. Advances in synthetic biology are about to enable a shorter time to development. Currently, virus production begins with the creation of a hybrid virus strain using classical genetics. Growth and isolation of a hybrid virus with the right mix of genes from two parental strains can take 35 days. Synthetic biologists have now developed a method to produce the exact virus needed for a vaccine in as few as five days. The key is rapid synthesis of a DNA copy of the influenza virus genome, which is transfected into mammalian cells to produce an actual virus.

Scientific opportunities and challenges

Advances in modern biology offer new solutions to some of the challenges posed by infectious diseases. In the near future, several developments in synthetic biology will likely lead to new approaches to prevent, mitigate, and control infectious diseases.

Low-cost synthetic DNA. Large DNA molecules, comprised of a few thousand nucleotide bases pairs to more than a million bases pairs, can currently be synthesized for about US$0.30 per base pair. In the near future, new technologies should decrease costs 10- to 100-fold. Similar increases in the speed of synthesis should also occur. Rapid, inexpensive gene and genome synthesis will enable faster exploration of new options for developing therapies.

Synthetic vaccinology. Synthetic biology is already being used to produce vaccines more rapidly. It also offers solutions to challenges associated with vaccine development, such as product safety concerns, cost and time to clinical development, and design of vaccines against pathogens with high and shifting antigenic diversity. Synthetic biology can be used to synthesize small influenza viral genomes and, more impressively, has been used to create a bacterial cell with a fully synthetic genome. Currently, developing and licensing a new vaccine can take decades and almost US$1 billion. However, using synthetic biology methods, it may be possible to create viral and bacterial vaccine platforms in which only the immunizing antigens are varied. Once a basic vaccine platform is approved by regulatory agencies, subsequent versions of vaccines created using that licensed platform could be approved via streamlined clinical trials and be made in existing manufacturing facilities. Many of the most intractable vaccine targets, such as HIV and rhinovirus, are characterized by overwhelming antigenic diversity. Synthetic biology gives us the possibility of making multivalent vaccines in which a single attenuated organism or virus can evoke the production of various antibodies.

New chemical libraries. Almost all drugs are derived from a natural source. These chemical drugs are synthesized by clusters of genes dedicated to the production of a specific chemical. Many of these chemicals are used by the organisms to wage war on their neighbors. One of the surprises of genome analysis is that for every gene cluster producing a known metabolite, microbes contain 10 other metabolic clusters that we do not know what their product would be. Presumably, these gene clusters produce their metabolite only under specific unknown conditions. Synthetic biologists are now resynthesizing the elements of these gene clusters with each gene under the control of inducible promoters (i.e., gene triggers). These synthetic DNA modules are then inserted into organisms (e.g., bacteria) and induced to express the natural product. This approach will produce libraries of natural products that can be screened for useful activity. These will likely be rich sources of new antibiotics and anti-cancer drugs.

Risks and concerns about synthetic biology. In our post 9/11 world, with the advent of synthetic biology came increased concerns about bioterrorism and lapses in laboratory safety. This was especially true after the JCVI's announcement that a synthetic bacterial cell had been made. Although the public and governmental organizations have expressed concerns that the synthetic cell technology would lead to bioterrorists creating new untreatable bacterial pathogens, currently this technology is too expensive and difficult to pose a significant risk. However, the technology enabling the JCVI to more rapidly produce influenza virus vaccines could also be used to make viral pathogens. Disturbingly, a virologist/synthetic biologist could create polio virus, a pathogen no longer commonly immunized against, for less than US$5,000.

Policy issues

- **Reform intellectual property incentives for creating new antibiotics.** The pharmaceutical industry has largely abandoned infectious diseases research, especially for those diseases that principally infect the poor. The prospect of antibiotic resistance limiting the profitability of a new drug before its patent expires is a disincentive for developing new antibiotics. Intellectual property reforms may require revision of the current approach to patents. In exchange for new antibiotic creation, especially for diseases of the poor such as TB, drug companies could be rewarded with patent extensions on existing nonantibiotic drugs aimed at more affluent populations.

- **Decrease the regulatory burden for drugs and vaccines made using recombinant DNA technology.** In the U.S. and many other countries, genetically modified organisms (GMOs) and products produced using such organisms are subject to more stringent regulations than organisms and products made without recombinant or synthetic DNA. The U.S. regulatory framework for GMOs, often involving multiple agencies, creates a disincentive to the use of this superior technology. Scientists need to explain to the public the relative risks of organisms produced using designed, as opposed to random (natural), mutations. The scientific community and policy makers in each nation should work together to develop consistent regulations.

- **Develop a scientifically literate public.** The anti-vaccine movement would not have found wide acceptance if society understood what constitutes scientific proof and had a basic knowledge about biology. It is the responsibility of policy makers, educators, and the scientific community to improve the public's scientific competence. Scientists should commit 1%–5% of their time educating the public and policy makers about science. This public education effort should be required of all scientific teams receiving public funding.
- **Require commercial DNA synthesizers to deny sale to unauthorized users of synthetic genes and oligonucleotides that could be used to synthesize pathogenic viruses and toxins.** Currently, some U.S. DNA producers screen orders to ensure that whole genes that could be used to make certain pathogens or toxin genes are not sold; however oligonucleotide orders that would enable pathogen or toxin synthesis should be screened as well. This should be a worldwide policy. Scientists, DNA manufacturers, and policy makers should convene to develop uniform policies in this regard. Permits to receive such DNA should go to certain groups.

** A policy position paper prepared for presentation at the conference on Emerging and Persistent Infectious Diseases (EPID): Focus on Mitigation convened by the Institute on Science for Global Policy (ISGP) Oct. 23–26, 2011, at the University of Edinburgh, Edinburgh, Scotland.

Debate Summary

The following summary is based on notes recorded by the ISGP staff during the not-for-attribution debate of the policy position paper prepared by Dr. John Glass (see above). Dr. Glass initiated the debate with a 5-minute statement of his views and then actively engaged the conference participants, including other authors, throughout the remainder of the 90-minute period. This Debate Summary represents the ISGP's best effort to accurately capture the comments offered and questions posed by all participants, as well as those responses made by Dr. Glass. Given the not-for-attribution format of the debate, the views comprising this summary do not necessarily represent the views of Dr. Glass, as evidenced by his policy position paper. Rather, it is, and should be read as, an overview of the areas of agreement and disagreement that emerged from all those participating in the critical debate.

Debate conclusions

- Compared to traditional molecular biology, technologies based on synthetic biology synthesize genes exponentially faster, and in significantly greater quantities, by creating biological organisms using only digital information and the appropriate chemicals. By providing an alternative to vaccine production via egg-based technologies and conventional pharmaceutical development, synthetic biology can have a significant positive impact on the prevention and mitigation of infectious diseases. Major changes in regulatory policies and procedures are required to support such novel uses of synthetic biology.

- Concern over the potential negative use of synthetic biology, both accidental and intentional, has motivated efforts to regulate access to databases, biological material, and the equipment associated with synthetic biology. Emphasis on the regulation of synthetic biology has intensified with the involvement of "do-it-yourselfers" and the potential involvement of bioterrorists.

- It is imperative to balance synthetic biology regulation with the flexibility required for scientific progress. There is a danger that over-regulation in certain parts of the world could stifle innovation, curb scientific competitiveness, and limit the ability to respond if a negative event arises related to synthetic biology.

- As with any potentially transformational technology, policy makers and the public need to acknowledge the inherent risks of synthetic biology without being overly alarmist. The history of genetically modified organisms (GMOs) in Europe, where their use is now severely limited, serves as a warning about the negative consequences that can occur when such debates are framed improperly and depart from scientifically credible information.

Current realities

The debate acknowledged the significant advances currently being made in the field of synthetic biology, which have already improved — and will likely continue to improve — infectious disease prevention and mitigation. The rapid growth in the application of synthetic biology to infectious diseases, as well as across a large number of fields (e.g., medicine, energy, and biomaterials) was highlighted. For example, through the implementation of new technologies created by synthetic biology, DNA sequences stored on computers can be used to rapidly and inexpensively produce actual DNA that can be incorporated into cells and viruses to endow them with properties that can aid in the development of medicines, vaccines, and other materials.

Synthetic biology, it was agreed, differs greatly from traditional molecular biology in terms of both the scale and speed with which new material can be created. It is now much easier, and exponentially faster, to make multiple variants of genes with automated methods using synthetic biology applications. For example, synthesis of DNA copies of influenza genes, which used to take weeks, can now be done within hours. Differing opinions were expressed as to whether synthetic biology is a "revolutionary" technology (i.e., a groundbreaking development that is qualitatively different from older technologies) or an "evolutionary" technology (i.e., an extension of existing fields such as molecular biology). It was contended that synthetic biology is "revolutionary" because unlike in molecular biology, where genetic engineering must start with a biological entity, it is possible to synthesize a genome and create an organism starting only with information on a computer database and the appropriate chemicals. Creating a virus such as polio, which would be extremely difficult in molecular biology, therefore becomes possible. Those who argued that it should be regarded as evolutionary countered that while the methods might be innovative, synthetic biology currently can only be used to create things that already exist. Although no consensus was reached about the extent to which synthetic biology can be regarded as "new," such debates were noted to have important implications for regulation.

Concern was raised about the potential for harmful consequences stemming from intentional or inadvertent misuse of synthetic biology tools. An amateur scientist or member of the public can access databases such as GenBank (an online database of all publicly available DNA sequences), download a series of specified oligonucleotide sequences, and then order DNA from a commercial DNA synthesizing company. However, it was emphasized that an extremely high level of expertise is still required to create a virulent pathogen. Since it is currently almost impossible to create a pathogen by accident because it is incredibly difficult to increase the pathogenicity of an organism, the most significant concern at present lies in the possibility of intentional misuse. It was argued that attempts will inevitably be made to use synthetic biology for nefarious purposes. Given conflicting arguments regarding the extent of the risks, it was generally agreed the risks are outweighed by the benefits and the perception that synthetic biology is more dangerous than previous genetic engineering projects does not reflect reality.

Great disparity worldwide in attitudes toward synthetic biology was noted. For example, while agencies in some less-affluent countries are reluctant to accept synthetically made vaccines, others such as the United States' National Institutes of Health (NIH) and Food and Drug Administration (FDA) are increasingly amenable to using such vaccines. Given progress in the acceptability of synthetic vaccines in countries like the U.S., it was noted that a major pharmaceutical company is preparing to produce synthetic influenza vaccines within the next few years.

Similarly, discussion focused on global disparities in the regulation of activities related to synthetic biology. Control of synthetic biology research was considered inconsistent throughout the world. While the U.S. and Europe are moving toward stricter regulation, other parts of the world presently have limited or even no guidelines or regulatory framework for the use of synthetic biology. The lack of an international regulatory framework to oversee this technology was repeatedly highlighted during the debate.

Scientific opportunities and challenges

Increased accessibility to a range of DNA sequence information was regarded as both an opportunity and a challenge. As gene synthesis becomes cheaper (currently it costs US$.07 per nucleotide base) and faster, synthetic biology will likely become accessible to scientists in increasingly diverse disciplines. As a result, synthetic biology can potentially have a significant positive impact, not only in the field of infectious diseases, but also across a variety of scientific disciplines and industries (e.g., material sciences and the energy sector). Greater accessibility, however, also increases the likelihood that an individual with harmful intentions will be able to capitalize on synthetic biology. Limiting the potential for adverse events has become a major challenge.

Challenges related to the increasing accessibility of sequence information were discussed in this regard. It is theoretically possible to order DNA online and then synthesize genes within a few weeks using machines that can be purchased on Web sites. Thus, the potential exists for scientists to create pathogens outside of a supervised laboratory. Technological improvements in the next few years likely will result in an increasing number of DNA supply companies selling high-quality oligonucleotides. This raised particular concerns because DNA synthesizing companies in the U.S. screen and monitor DNA sequence orders for potential toxins or viruses, but orders for oligonucleotides are not usually screened.

Harm from synthetic biology-related activities could potentially result from: (i) accidental misuse, (ii) the activities of a rogue scientist or "Do-It-Yourselfer," or (iii) terrorist activities. Those who were uneasy about the possibility of accidental misuse highlighted the considerable independence afforded to those students taking part in the International Genetically Engineered Machine Competition (iGEM). Others countered that it is extremely difficult to unwittingly increase the pathogenicity of an organism or, in fact, maintain pathogenicity at all. Thus, malicious intent was generally considered a much likelier potential hazard than accidental mishap. The increasing availability of DNA, oligonucleotides, and synthetic biology tools raised concerns about rogue, "maladjusted" scientists. Even with stringent regulation, it was seen as impossible to rule out the chance of someone creating a harmful pathogen. By way of analogy, prohibition in the U.S. did not prevent the production of alcohol. Bioterrorism was also deemed a threat, because full international control over synthetic biology activity is considered unfeasible.

However, there was little consensus regarding the general extent of the risks associated with synthetic biology. It was noted that since the 1975 Asilomar Conference on Recombinant DNA, where dire predictions were made about the effect that genetic engineering might have on society, there has not yet been a single incident in which synthetic biology applications have caused a significant negative impact. This was countered, however, by those who argued that recent advances in synthetic biology will likely create risks that we have not yet had to face.

There was consensus that the scientific capability to predict exact phenotypes, via reverse genetics, of viruses reconstructed or generated through synthetic biology does not currently exist. This was considered a challenge in terms of biosecurity.

The question was raised as to whether it is possible to create monitoring technology that would enable the tracing of engineered or synthetic organisms in the event of an accidental or intentional release. While it is currently possible to "sign" work so that it can be traced to its original owner, determining how to persuade synthetic biologists to always use these tags or tracers, especially if they have malicious intent, remained an unresolved issue.

It was noted that it is possible to contain engineered organisms by altering their genetic code to require a synthetic amino acid for protein synthesis. Requiring an engineered organism to use an altered amino acid, not available in nature, will theoretically render it unable to survive outside of controlled laboratory conditions. While scientists believe that these controlled organisms are unlikely to survive outside the laboratory, it cannot be guaranteed that this will always be the case. It was similarly argued that it is impossible to prevent organisms designed to create positive outcomes from entering the environment and causing unintentional harm due to unpredictable genetic changes. The development of effective safety mechanisms would minimize the risk of adverse outcomes, even if these risks cannot be completely eliminated.

Synthetic biology was seen as a tool that is creating important opportunities for influenza mitigation. For instance, synthetic biology enables the production of influenza vaccines in mammalian cells instead of chicken eggs. This methodology dramatically reduces the length of the first stage of the vaccine production process from approximately 35 days to five days. Additionally, scientists can monitor and synthesize millions of different strains of influenza viruses simultaneously. In doing so, a vaccine can be produced quickly to counter a specific virus recognized to have pandemic potential. This reduction in production time would ensure that a greater number of people are vaccinated before they are exposed to the disease. During the 2009 H1N1 outbreak, it was noted that the pandemic had already peaked by the time a vaccine was created using then-current production methods. Had H1N1 been more virulent, morbidity and mortality would have been considerably higher. However, vaccine production time is only one factor determining vaccine availability; scientific advancements that can speed up production do not affect other hurdles that vaccines must go through (e.g., testing, the regulatory process). It was argued that in theory, testing and regulatory approval could also be significantly accelerated.

Differences were highlighted in the acceptance of synthetic vaccines throughout the world. While some countries in Europe currently market influenza vaccines that have been synthetically created in mammalian cells, this is not universally accepted throughout the continent. Additionally, in some parts of the world, such as in Africa, government channels are more wary of — and do not currently want — any genetically modified organism as a vaccine. It was speculated that such dismissive views could change in the near future.

There were questions regarding the likelihood that a synthetic vaccine would be approved by the FDA. Although support for certain synthetic vaccines is believed to be growing in the U.S., it was acknowledged that several hurdles will need to be crossed before a synthetic vaccine can pass the FDA's regulatory process. In theory, the process for synthetic vaccine approval could be sped significantly. Yet, it was acknowledged this would only happen if there was political will to do so.

It was suggested that synthetic biology be used to develop a combined diagnostic/vaccine system, which would make it possible to detect the difference between vaccinated and infected animals. This would potentially prevent the need for large-scale animal slaughter in the case of an epidemic. During the foot-and-mouth outbreak in the United Kingdom, many animals were unnecessarily slaughtered because technology that could separate healthy animals from those that were infected was not available. While there was general agreement that a combined diagnostic/vaccine system would be useful, scientists do not yet possess the biological knowledge that would enable them to create such a product.

It was noted that one of the most important challenges is that biological understanding lags behind technical expertise. Thus, while scientists know how to create sequences, *what* to make is often unknown. For example, vaccine production to prevent certain viruses (e.g., influenza, polio, smallpox) is simple; however, for organisms with complicated "handshakes" with the immune system, the development of new vaccines is extremely difficult.

Policy issues

The risk of inadvertent or deliberate harm resulting from synthetic biology-related activities, such as the possibility of the intentional or accidental creation of bacterial pathogens, warrants careful and precautionary guidelines and regulation. Although it was acknowledged that it is extremely difficult to increase the pathogenicity of a genome with current technology, it was countered that a regulatory framework is required to mitigate the potential risk of bioterrorism in the future. While prominent bodies are recognizing the need for regulation (e.g., in a 2004 Institute of Medicine report), many governments have been slow to act on these issues. One specific area where the need for regulation was emphasized related to screening: a screening system is needed that blocks people from ordering DNA agents that could be used to make potentially dangerous viruses or organisms.

While sentiments promoting the development and implementation of new regulations were voiced, it was argued that additional regulatory mechanisms are not necessary. Regulations were seen as already in place to handle GMOs, which can be applied to synthetic biology. Synthetic biology, it was argued, is not sufficiently different from GMOs (except for scale and pace) to warrant new, additional regulations. However, there were concerns that the crippling effect that stringent European regulations have had on the use of GMOs in many parts of Europe would be repeated for synthetic biology. Regardless of whether GMO regulations are used as a model, even if regulations existed, intentional harm caused by terrorists or a "lone operator" would not necessarily be halted. The possibility for abusing technology will always exist. Another critique of implementing new regulations was that the potential harm of synthetic biology is overstated.

The potentially negative implications of regulations were also raised as an obstacle to be considered before such policies are instituted. Implementing new regulations could excessively heighten perceptions of the dangers associated with synthetic biology, which may impede public acceptance of such technologies. There was general agreement that it is imperative that innovation is not unduly stifled. Some regulations were seen as making it more difficult for scientists to do their work. For example, in Europe, regulation has impeded GMO technology for the past 15 years. However, it was countered that regulations are not necessarily an impediment to progress, and that many scientists are willing to accept regulations as a precondition of conducting the science.

Varying regulations throughout the world were seen as creating a disadvantage for the countries and regions that institute more stringent rules. For example, the Obama Administration Bioethics Report concluded being "ahead of the game" is the best way to address a terrorist threat and manage the consequences of terrorists' use of synthetic biology to create a disease. Regulations applied only to laboratories in some countries and regions (e.g., the U.S. and Europe) may impede these countries' ability to conduct the necessary research to be prepared in the event of a bioterrorist incident. If more-affluent countries increasingly regulate emerging technologies, while the rest of the world does not, it was noted the development and advancement of science and technology in wealthier countries may lag behind other regions.

Alternatives to strong government regulation or the formation of a new governmental regulatory body were sought. It was proposed that the implementation of a "gentle structure" might sufficiently negate the need for a governmental body, although the components of such a structure were not defined. To control the potential ramifications of this technology, it was contended that regulation be one part of a multifaceted approach that also includes an informal code of conduct for scientists.

Regulation in other arenas, such as nuclear activities or computer viruses, was seen as a potential model for regulating synthetic biology activities. Regulation in these areas has often reflected cooperation between the private and public sectors (e.g., in terms of tracing hacking) and has demonstrated positive exchanges of information and intelligence across different agencies. It was countered that synthetic biology has sufficiently distinct risks and therefore warrants its own unique regulatory actions.

It was noted there is increasing awareness of the need for self-regulation within the field of synthetic biology. For example, the International Association of Synthetic Biology (IASB) subscribes to a code system for DNA suppliers and plans to discuss expanding the code system to customers and the research community next year. Additionally, at iGEM Asia, participating competitors had to include implications for biosafety and biosecurity in their project proposals. It was proposed that informal systems already in place within the field of synthetic biology, such as the International Gene Synthesis Consortium (IGSC) in the U.S., be formalized and provided with support.

It was contended that intellectual property regulation was missing from the discussion. Particularly given that it is unchartered territory for synthetic biology, intellectual property regulation was seen as a concern for the scientific community. Countering this view was the suggestion that there be no regulation in the intellectual property realm because the information should be available to all who are "fit" to use it.

Educating current and future scientists was seen as a potentially constructive way to prevent intentional or unintentional harm from occurring through synthetic biology activities. It was suggested that a substantial part of graduate education for those who work in synthetic biology-related technologies include understanding their responsibilities, the risks involved, and their obligations to the field and to society. Some universities are already incorporating this type of education into their curricula.

Because of the global dissemination of synthetic biology-related technologies, it was argued that the public must be educated about the risks and benefits of the field. Scientists were cautioned against overemphasizing the risks of synthetic biology. While negative perceptions and misunderstandings of risks may be difficult to correct, scientific advancement is often suppressed when such views are not countered. The example provided was of the European public's attitude against GMOs, which, it was asserted, limited their use in the region.

Innovation, Policy, and Public Interactions in the Management of Infectious Diseases**

Joyce Tait, C.B.E., F.R.S.E., D. Univ. (Open), Ph.D., B.Sc.
Professor and Scientific Advisor, Innogen Centre, University of Edinburgh

Summary

This paper focuses on preparedness planning for an influenza pandemic, particularly the impact of specific policies on national health-related and economic outcomes. The case fatality rate (CFR) of a new influenza strain is likely to be the primary determinant of public behavior, leading to actions including individuals absenting themselves from work due to fear of infection (i.e., prophylactic absenteeism [PA]). Such behaviors impact the effectiveness of preparedness plans. Synthetic biology is a promising approach for the rapid development of improved diagnostics and vaccines, with enormous potential savings to national economies. Regulatory innovations are needed to enable rapid development of these technologies to address the emergence of a new pandemic strain of influenza. Throughout this paper, the United Kingdom is used to exemplify preparedness planning in a real-world setting. Similar points would apply to any other country operating, or planning to operate, a similar system of contingency planning and decision-making.

Current realities

The emergence in East Asia of a new strain of H5N1 avian influenza at the end of the 20th century has been a major concern among health authorities globally because, although it is only rarely transmitted to humans, it has a very high CFR. If it should mutate to a form that can readily infect humans while retaining this high CFR, it could cause a global pandemic of potentially devastating proportions. National and international health authorities have been developing preparedness plans for addressing the H5N1 threat since before 2005. Thus, in 2009, the unexpected emergence of an H1N1 strain of the influenza virus (frequently referred to as "swine flu") encountered a relatively well-prepared response. Indeed, given that the CFR of the new H1N1 strain turned out to be low, the response provided a useful test of these preparedness plans in a context where any weaknesses that were revealed did not result in serious health or economic outcomes.

Preparedness planning in the U.K. is based on two largely irreconcilable objectives: minimizing direct health impacts and minimizing the indirect impact on the economy. Policies to achieve the first of these objectives include actions such as closing schools and more general "social distancing" (i.e., encouraging the public to avoid crowded places and prolonged contact with large numbers of people). On the other hand, policies to achieve the economic objective, described as "business as usual," encourage uninfected people to behave normally (e.g., going to work). These two key objectives thus result in ambiguity in official advice in the event of a pandemic. Figure 1 explores potential economic outcomes from the tension between these two objectives, and examines perceived weaknesses in specific parts of the preparedness planning system related to factors such as risk communication, maintaining transport systems, delivery of food and fuel, coping with the demands on the health care system to diagnose disease, and delivery of drugs and vaccines.

Public response in the early stages of the 2009 H1N1 pandemic, before it was clear that the CFR was similar to a normal winter influenza epidemic, suggests that serious flaws in current preparedness plans would have been magnified if the H1N1 CFR had been higher. For example, there was evidence of some panic buying of drugs, stockpiling of face masks, and healthy people absenting themselves from work because of PA. There was also considerable controversy and some confusion around decisions to close some schools.

Based on the scenario in Figure 1, and building on standard epidemiological and U.K.-based economic modeling, an analysis was conducted to determine the potential impact of various combinations of mortality and morbidity from influenza, vaccine efficacy, school closures, and PA on the U.K. economy (Smith et al., 2009). The analysis found that the costs related to illness alone ranged between 0.5% and 1.0% of the gross domestic product (GDP) (UK£8.4 billion to UK£16.8 billion) for low-fatality scenarios, 3.3% and 4.3% (UK£55.5 billion to UK£72.3 billion) for high fatality scenarios, and larger still for an extreme pandemic with a CFR of up to 10% (e.g., as was the case for SARS). School closure increased the economic impact, particularly for mild pandemics, but had only a modest impact on infection rates. Vaccination with a pre-pandemic vaccine was calculated to save 0.13% to 2.3% of GDP (UK£2.2 billion to UK£38.6 billion); a single dose of a matched vaccine could save 0.3% to 4.3% (UK£5.0 billion to UK£72.3 billion); and two doses of a matched vaccine could limit the overall economic impact to about 1% of GDP for all disease scenarios.

One of the main drivers of economic impact in any pandemic is likely to be PA, assumed to be driven by the size of the CFR rather than by the infection rate, related to having an acquaintance die from the disease (the threshold being a CFR of 2.5%–5%). In this analysis, the impact of PA on the economy was more than quadruple the effect of the aforementioned factors. Even without PA, vaccine development and production will likely result in economic savings that outweigh the cost. The additional role of vaccination in providing reassurance and reducing the extent of PA will also greatly magnify these benefits.

Scientific opportunities and challenges

The above factors place a high premium on faster development of disease diagnostics (to characterize the nature of the organism for an emerging infectious disease and to distinguish infected from uninfected individuals) and on vaccines (to reduce both the infection rate and the extent of PA). Synthetic biology — combining large-scale DNA sequencing, artificial gene synthesis, and vaccine development using synthetically produced antigens — could allow for the rapid deployment of a new vaccine in response to a novel infection outbreak, as in the recent H1N1 influenza outbreak (Burbelo et al., 2010).

Artificial gene synthesis offers a shortcut to immunoassay development to detect human antibodies with high levels of sensitivity and specificity, resulting in a better diagnostic performance than natural proteins and increasing the spectrum and quality of immunodiagnostics. One technique is to generate a repeating peptide in a single protein to develop antibody-based tests for antigens, which leads to improved diagnostic performance compared to testing individual, natural, strain-specific proteins.

In vaccine development, bioinformatics can be used for engineering artificial proteins that match highly complex antigenic strain variations to induce a greater immune response. Two promising techniques currently in development are: 1) the creation of bioengineered antigens representing diverse strains of an organism to provide broad vaccine protection and 2) the use of synthetic attenuated viral engineering to produce live vaccines (modified viruses with proteomes identical to the virulent one, but with less than optimal codons and codon pairs, which render the pathogenic viruses unable to grow or replicate efficiently and allow the infected host to mount a powerful immune response against the weakened virus). Synthetic biology will also have a role in the engineering of microorganisms for more rapid large-scale manufacture of these novel vaccines.

Policy issues

Planning for civil contingencies, including pandemic preparedness, aims to integrate the maintenance of key public services (e.g., health care, schooling, food distribution, transport, energy provision, banking), based on encouragement of community resilience and plans for maintenance of law and order. As noted above and in Figure 1, this will require an unprecedented degree of national-level policy collaboration, based on a good understanding of likely human behavior in response to a pandemic; there is room for improvement in both of these areas. In addition, the ability of synthetic biology to deliver better diagnostics and vaccines more quickly will require matching policy innovation at national and international levels to facilitate more rapid regulatory approval of these tools (EMA, 2011). Policy developments in civil contingency planning and product regulation will provide the physical and biological tools to minimize the health impacts of a pandemic or epidemic and will create an optimal societal environment for their application.

- *A coordinated national socioeconomic research strategy* is needed, well informed by an understanding of disease processes and of relevant scientific developments, to improve understanding of the likely behavior of members of the public and of official and unofficial responders in a range of pandemic scenarios. One outcome of this should be improved public communication plans based on the insights gained. **Proposed leads:** government research funders.

- *An open and robust planning and communication strategy for pandemic preparedness planning* must be developed that takes account of the views of those who will implement the plans, considers the outcomes of the socioeconomic analyses recommended above, and is able to integrate regional and local plans at a national level within clear and workable decision-making structures (including decision-making frameworks and designated decision-making powers). **Proposed leads:** local, regional, and national government officials across all functions involved in addressing a pandemic.

- *A science and innovation strategy* should be created and implemented to build on developments in synthetic biology to develop better methods for rapid characterization of novel disease organisms and more rapid development of effective vaccines matched to these organisms. **Proposed leads:** government bodies that fund basic science and medical science research.

- *Policy innovation* to support more rapid passage of new diagnostics and vaccines through safety and efficacy testing, including development of new, improved approaches to safety and efficacy testing (potentially also based on synthetic biology) and appropriate revisions of policy processes. **Proposed leads:** the U.S. Food and Drug Administration (FDA), the European Medicines Agency (EMA), and national regulators.

References

Burbelo, P. D., Ching, K. H., Han, B. L., Klimavicz, C. M., & Iadarola, M. J. (2010). Synthetic biology for translational research. *American Journal of Translational Research, 2(4)*, 381-389.

European Medicines Agency (EMA). (2011, April). *Pandemic report and lessons learned: Outcome of the European Medicines Agency's activities during the 2009 (H1N1) flu pandemic.* (EMA/221017/2011). Retrieved August 7, 2011, from http: www.ema.europa. eu/docs/en_GB/document_library/Report/2011/04/WC500105820.pdf.

Smith R. D., Keogh-Brown, M. R., Barnett, T., & Tait, J. (2009). The economy-wide impact of pandemic influenza on the UK: A computable general equilibrium modelling experiment. *BMJ, 339*, b4571.

*** A policy position paper prepared for presentation at the conference on Emerging and Persistent Infectious Diseases (EPID): Focus on Mitigation convened by the Institute on Science for Global Policy (ISGP) Oct. 23–26, 2011, at the University of Edinburgh, Edinburgh, Scotland.*

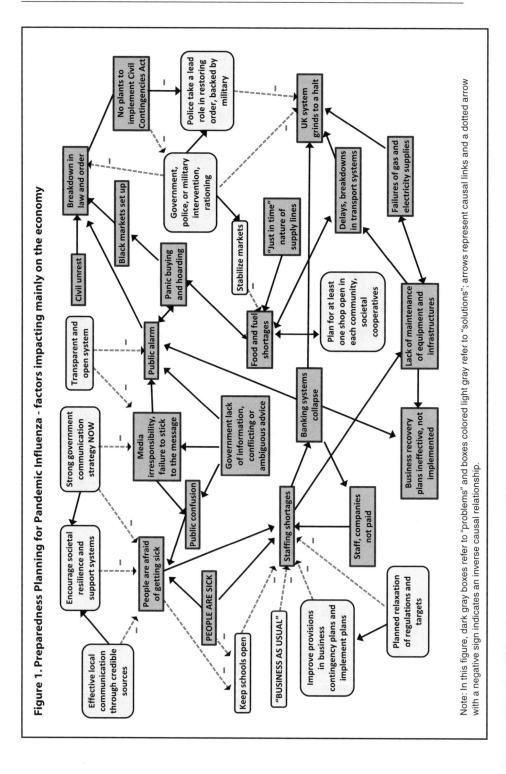

Figure 1. Preparedness Planning for Pandemic Influenza - factors impacting mainly on the economy

Note: In this figure, dark gray boxes refer to "problems" and boxes colored light gray refer to "solutions"; arrows represent causal links and a dotted arrow with a negative sign indicates an inverse causal relationship.

Debate Summary

The following summary is based on notes recorded by the ISGP staff during the not-for-attribution debate of the policy position paper prepared by Prof. Joyce Tait (see above). Prof. Tait initiated the debate with a 5-minute statement of her views and then actively engaged the conference participants, including other authors, throughout the remainder of the 90-minute period. This Debate Summary represents the ISGP's best effort to accurately capture the comments offered and questions posed by all participants, as well as those responses made by Prof. Tait. Given the not-for-attribution format of the debate, the views comprising this summary do not necessarily represent the views of Prof. Tait, as evidenced by her policy position paper. Rather, it is, and should be read as, an overview of the areas of agreement and disagreement that emerged from all those participating in the critical debate.

Debate conclusions

- There is conflicting evidence on the effectiveness of some interventions that have been implemented to mitigate the spread of influenza, such as social distancing measures (including school closures) and face masks. Conflicting evidence about infectious disease mitigation approaches has led to differential policies throughout the world, and sometimes, contradictory and ambiguous guidance within countries. Improved research (e.g., cluster randomized trials) is needed to better understand intervention effectiveness.

- Ambiguity in contingency planning advice is exemplified by some governments simultaneously asking the public to conduct "business as usual" to minimize a pandemic's economic impact, and guiding people to use precautionary social distancing (e.g., staying away from work even if they are not sick) to minimize a pandemic's health impact. There is a need to determine which benchmarks (e.g., case fatality rates [CFRs]) can be used to transition between an emphasis on economic- versus health-motivated recommendations to the public.

- To be effective, contingency planning must consider ways to limit the individual-level economic ramifications of infectious disease mitigation efforts. Social distancing guidance is hindered in countries where work policies do not protect or compensate nonsalaried individuals when they are absent from work due to illness. Policies need to plan for the no-show and/or desertion rate of workers during a pandemic, which may cause food and cash shortages, lack of transportation, and health care system breakdowns.

- The media must be proactively incorporated into the public messaging used for mitigating infectious disease pandemics. Educating the media concerning the accuracy of messages to the public can be critical in the contingency planning for pandemics. As information changes, public health officials need to effectively communicate new instructions to the public without reducing public confidence in the competency of authorities.

- Vaccines not only have demonstrated health benefits, but also support economies by limiting precautionary social distancing when workers are assured it is safe to work or travel. Significant barriers to rapid vaccine development and distribution remain (e.g., the scientific challenges of bulk manufacturing, financial reluctance to large-scale manufacturing because of funding uncertainties, regulatory roadblocks). Vaccine development and distribution processes need to be accelerated using innovative approaches including research such as the identification of common influenza virus vaccines (i.e., effective against all strains) as well as proactive policies that incentivize regulatory bodies and their pharmaceutical counterparts.

Current realities

A large part of the discussion centered on the successes and challenges related to the 2009 "swine" influenza pandemic (PDM 2009 H1N1) mitigation effort. There were sharply divided opinions on whether the planning for, and response to, the PDM 2009 H1N1 pandemic was successful overall. It was clear, however, that there were components of the mitigation effort that worked well and others that did not work as well.

While it was recognized that improvements could have been made in the planning for and mitigation of the PDM 2009 H1N1 pandemic, several specific successes in the United States were identified that are now influencing current planning. Regional planning was strengthened, as indicated by new liaisons with Canada and Mexico. Public messaging was also identified as having been improved as illustrated by three clear, consistent messages (i.e., cover your cough, stay home if you are sick, wash your hands), publicly conveyed through conduits such as videos. In addition, communication about travel was noted as being excellent. The improved ability in sharing messages was subsequently applied to travel messaging in the wake of the Fukushima nuclear disaster in Japan.

In terms of vaccines, H1N1 was noted as an extraordinary success story for technology because a vaccine was available within five months. Furthermore, hospitals mandated influenza vaccinations for health care providers. Rapid distribution of vaccines in the U.S., especially into schools, was an example of success that demonstrated the benefits of proactive planning. Specific advances in vaccines for H1N1 were highlighted, including reductions in sterility testing times.

Criticisms of, and challenges with, PDM 2009 H1N1 mitigation efforts were also identified. The government response was not scaled appropriately and critical parts of the infrastructure needed for vaccination and treatment were not given high priority. These failings were attributed in part to planning based too heavily on 1918 influenza pandemic scenarios. Convincing people to stay home when sick was also identified as an unresolved challenge, especially because many people do not get paid when they are absent from work for any reason.

It was argued that mitigation efforts appeared successful primarily because the CFR was lower than originally expected and that, if the rate had been higher, infrastructure systems would have broken down and the mitigation efforts would have failed.

Scientific opportunities and challenges

Among the many lessons learned from the PDM 2009 H1N1 pandemic, much of the debate focused on quarantine and social distancing interventions. Of note, discussion centered on the advice concerning school closures and guidance for individuals to stay home from work and other public places (e.g., public transportation) if they are sick. The extent to which such interventions are effective remains to be determined because of contradictory research findings. Some data show that social distancing is not effective. For example, during the PDM 2009 H1N1 pandemic, continued use of public transport and work attendance did not have a notable impact on the infection rate; in addition, a recent Cochrane collaboration found only marginal benefits of social distancing. Conversely, examples of successful effects of social distancing interventions in some countries (e.g., Mexico) were found. There is also conflicting evidence regarding school closures. Both published and unpublished research has documented the effectiveness of school closures in countries including Canada, France, and Japan. However, other studies have shown that school closings had a very small impact on the level of infection in the PDM 2009 H1N1 pandemic and, in addition, were disruptive to families. Further, it was argued that the decrease in influenza transmission, which coincided with school summer breaks, had more to do with the winter seasonality of influenza than school closures.

When children stay home from school, but then go to public places (e.g., museums or shopping malls), the benefits of distancing may be negated. Anecdotal data shows that what families choose to do when their children are not in school depends on factors such as the complexity of family structure and location. Further, an indirect negative implication of social distancing was highlighted: The more effective social distancing is demonstrated to be, the more likely it is that a "runaway precautionary social distancing problem" will occur that will create societal disruption during a pandemic. The implementation and thus, effectiveness, of school closings, depends on the CFR; a high CFR may influence parents to keep their children at home and not associate with other children.

School closures also frequently cause parents to stay home to care for their children. Because child rearing tends to be primarily women's responsibility, and women comprise the majority of the health care work force in some regions (e.g., the U.K.), school closures may have a major impact on the health care system's ability to address a pandemic. Data from private industry could provide important information on the economic impact (e.g., through the absence of workers) of interventions such as school closures, though it was acknowledged that industries may not want to advertise this vulnerability.

Much of the confusion and conflicting views about the effectiveness of social distancing may be due to poorly designed studies on social distancing itself, as well as public health myths surrounding this type of intervention. Some studies may underestimate the effect of social distancing interventions because, in the case of school closings, for example, children may not truly be "socially distanced" if they engage in other activities outside their homes. Improved design of such studies is needed to isolate the quarantining and social distancing aspects by controlling factors known to impact infection (e.g., hand washing). Specifically, there was a call for cluster randomized trials instead of additional observational studies.

It was asserted that the U.K. government has provided ambiguous advice related to national contingency planning. While the government may try to minimize the economic impact of a pandemic by asking the public to conduct "business as usual," its announced goal may also focus on minimizing the pandemic's health impact by advising social distancing (i.e., that individuals should stay home if they are sick and to avoid getting sick).

Potential downstream impacts of people missing work were identified: supermarket shelves may empty; bank cash dispensing machines may not be serviced; and transportation systems may break down. Of note, however, if fewer people are going to work then there would be a lower demand in some areas (e.g., on the transport system).

It is not well understood which individuals (e.g., medical workers) would likely continue working in the case of a pandemic or biological incident, and therefore it was suggested that research is needed in this area. Based on research and anecdotal evidence from prior crisis situations (e.g., Hurricane Katrina, an outbreak of viral encephalitis infection among children in a hospital in Spain), the no-show and/or desertion rate of workers may be a sizable proportion of the work force. One seldom-considered issue is that many people will ensure the safety of their families before returning to work.

Because people do not always behave as expected, it was seen as imperative to determine the range of potential behaviors the public may exhibit during a pandemic to ensure adequate preparation for both likely and unlikely events. For example, in some areas, PDM 2009 H1N1 was predicted to affect rural children much later than children in urban areas. However, this lag did not occur because rural families had more frequent contact with urban areas than originally realized. Cultural factors impact behavior as well, and need to be considered. The CFR was argued to be a key factor in moderating behavior during a pandemic and, thus, the effectiveness of interventions.

There was some conflicting evidence about the effectiveness of face masks, which seemed to vary by country. These differences may be due to the type of mask, societal expectations, and other factors. For example, some British research showed that face masks are not effective for stopping influenza transmission, while Japanese data shows that wearing a mask is effective. Of note, face masks purchased over-the-counter at pharmaceutical shops or chemists were said to be ineffective and effective antiviral masks were said to be costly.

Vaccines were believed to provide value to the economy because they limit precautionary social distancing by assuring people it is safe to work or travel. It was argued that the economic benefit of using a vaccine as a precautionary measure may even be greater than the benefit of using the vaccine to mitigate the health impact of the disease, especially when a disease has a high CFR. It was asserted that these economic benefits justify a large financial and time commitment to the development of vaccines and modification of the regulatory system.

There are many steps to vaccine development and distribution, each of which may speed or slow the process. Even with new technologies and streamlined regulatory systems, there was disagreement regarding how quickly a vaccine could be produced and distributed in the event of a pandemic. It was agreed that the approval process can be fast-tracked, as has been previously demonstrated. For example, the European Commission and the European Medicines Agency were able to provide virtually instantaneous approval for the PDM 2009 H1N1 influenza vaccine because many key agencies and companies (including the pharmaceutical industry and World Health Organization [WHO]) had worked out an action plan in preparation for H5N1, as well as the fact that PDM 2009 H1N1 was treated as a strain change of influenza and not a novel pathogen. However, even in cases where approval of a vaccine can be fast-tracked, other barriers to vaccine development and distribution exist.

The time frame of vaccine delivery was considered primarily dependent on bulk manufacturing at a commercial scale. There was extended discussion regarding whether the barriers to faster bulk manufacture are purely biological or whether political and economic factors also come into play. While rapid bulk manufacture may be scientifically feasible, the process is lengthy because it is difficult to persuade pharmaceutical companies to manufacture on a large scale when there is uncertainty about whether governments would pay for the vaccine in primary or secondary care systems. While biological barriers to rapid bulk manufacture may be addressed by the use of synthetic biology techniques, at present, synthetic biology can only be used to decrease the initial vaccine development process from approximately 35 days to between 0–5 days.

It was suggested that the regulatory system could create incentives that would accelerate the development of vaccines. Many examples exist in other areas of technology in which market regulatory incentives stimulated innovation. For example, in California, regulations were implemented stating that after 10 years, all cars sold must emit less than 50% of the current emissions levels. Initially, the car manufacturers said this was not possible; however, once the guaranteed market was created and they did the research, they were in fact able to do this in five years.

One solution proposed to speed up the vaccine process was the development of a common influenza vaccine, effective against all strains. It was asserted that there is progress in this vein for HIV, and this approach may be transferrable to the influenza virus. This possibility is being investigated by major pharmaceutical companies.

Policy issues

Conflicting evidence about interventions to mitigate pandemics has led to differential policies throughout the world and sometimes contradictory and ambiguous guidance within countries. For example, in the U.K., the public was told that face masks were not effective and, thus, were not widely available. At the same time, face masks were made available to health care workers who are regularly exposed to infection. In addition, contradictory messages are amplified by the international nature of the media. In countries where public guidance does not suggest the use of face masks, seeing pictures of people in other countries wearing masks can lead to confusion. Ambiguous messages have the potential to create public alarm and suspicion. Nuances in the evidence also may not be incorporated into public guidance. For example, different masks have differential effectiveness; it was argued that this distinction is often not conveyed to the public.

The issue of who is responsible for decisions to implement interventions, such as social distancing measures (e.g., school closures), was identified as another complexity in pandemic planning. For example, in the U.K., decisions to close the schools are made by the school's head teacher and there is no legal basis by which the U.K. government could require a school to close or stay open. Although the legal basis for social distancing via school closures was not available to the U.K. government, this was ultimately not to be a major problem as regulations on student-teacher ratios meant that once a certain number of teachers were absent, schools were required to close without intervention.

It was questioned whether there is a CFR benchmark that can be identified to indicate when chaos would develop and public health responses may no longer be effective, possibly leading to the declaration of martial law. It may be impossible to predict the CFR that would lead to chaos, and it was not clear under what conditions martial law might, or could, be imposed. There is wide variation in crisis responses across countries. In the U.S., for example, governors have the authority to ask the National Guard to implement a mandatory quarantine; a similarly intricate process happens in the U.K.

Hospital response capacities also need to be determined. Factors such as how many patients or, potentially, dead bodies, a hospital can handle need to be examined. Other issues that may lead to chaos include the fact that hospital staff may not come to work for various reasons, including school closings, which may cause those staff members to stay home with their children.

The role of social class interacts with countries' policies to determine whether social distancing interventions (e.g., telling people to stay home from work if they are sick) can be implemented effectively. In the U.S., for example, it is not uncommon for people at all levels to be hourly workers with no holiday time, sick leave, or time off in general. It was cautioned that it is a major challenge, at least in the U.S., to get hourly, non-salaried workers to stay home from work since they will not be compensated. Published research shows that the number of days people are willing to stay home from work is directly related to their income: the lower the income the fewer days workers are willing to stay home.

While much of the social distancing discussions focused on school closings and work absenteeism, the point was raised that global policy related to social distancing needs to be addressed. It was asserted that placing social distancing in a global context for international policy is complex. For example, it is difficult to determine what to do about passengers who have been to a country with an endemic disease. Policies that need to be discussed further include country-to-country agreements, travel restrictions, and the international transport of cargo.

The use and timing of different types of interventions were discussed. It was questioned whether medical interventions (e.g., vaccines, therapeutics, and diagnostics) and nonmedical approaches (e.g., social distancing, masks) are complimentary, or whether one is more important than the other. It was also questioned whether implementing nonmedical approaches such as social distancing might provide time to develop and distribute vaccines, or if it is imperative to get vaccines developed and distributed as quickly as possible to avoid using social distancing. The specific combination of nonmedical and medical approaches used was considered to be country-specific, society-specific, and disease-specific. The point was raised that a one-size-fits-all policy would likely not work in all countries, because of factors such as disparate health care systems.

The media, it was agreed, must be proactively incorporated into the solution set for pandemic planning and mitigation. Accurate communication with the public — explaining how a pandemic would be addressed — must occur before a pandemic begins. While it was acknowledged that it is challenging to get people to pay attention when there is not a crisis, attempts to accurately communicate must be made. Once a pandemic occurs, communication may lead to "social amplification," which would be counterproductive. Including the media in these anticipatory plans can improve the effectiveness of the public messages as a key component of contingency planning for pandemics. Public health officials must find ways to communicate with the public as information changes, without reducing public confidence in the competency of authorities.

Contingency plans that incorporate communication strategies to counter mistrust in public health agencies or international organizations caused by mistakes or events were recommended. For example, mistrust may be created when a group with knowledge or power receives different vaccination guidance than the general public. One example cited was an incident in which physicians chose not to be vaccinated because they believed the vaccine could be harmful to them. Another example was a country in which the politicians and members of the army received a different type of influenza vaccine than was offered to the general public. Although the reason behind differential guidance was only due to contractual issues and varied sources of the vaccines, conspiracy theories developed, creating mistrust.

Leadership at all levels — government, communities, and homes — was identified as important in ensuring the effective implementation of interventions (e.g., social distancing). While government leadership was agreed to be a necessity, it was argued that solutions should include empowering people and communities to take responsibility for their own health and welfare, and to be a part of working toward a solution.

It was suggested that policy makers focus on identifying the exact point at which they will make the transition from advising "business as usual" to guiding people to use precautionary social distancing (e.g., staying away from work even if they are not sick). While this point depends on the CFR, there is no particular CFR identified for making such decisions. When the CFR is unknown, policy makers tend to maintain a precautionary attitude.

Prioritization for vaccinations — who will be vaccinated first in the case of a pandemic — was discussed. Preventive measures such as vaccines are typically provided first to high-risk groups facing the most severe reactions from the disease. An alternative approach, supported by emerging data, is for transmission groups to be vaccinated first. In addition to prioritizing the people who are most likely to spread the disease and who are the most vulnerable, it was asserted that health care workers should also be considered high priority. In the case of PDM 2009 H1N1 in the U.K., higher-risk groups were prioritized and while doctors were offered the vaccine they generally did not accept it.

It was agreed that mitigation is most difficult for the countries that first encounter an epidemic. These countries with a new (or re-emerging) outbreak are prone to making poor decisions regarding mitigating the epidemic. It was recommended that a team be created comprised of experts who know how to address an epidemic, and who would be available to come into a country by day three and train key decision makers in how to handle the epidemic, including what messages to send. The team would need knowledge and expertise about the particular elements that a country (particularly a developing country) with an unusual outbreak could institute to mitigate an epidemic.

Biographical Information of Scientific Presenters

Prof. Sir Roy Anderson, F.R.S., F.Med.Sci.

Prof. Sir Roy Anderson is Professor of Infectious Disease Epidemiology at Imperial College, University of London. He recently spent three years on secondment as Chief Scientific Adviser to the U.K. Ministry of Defence, returning to Imperial in 2007. Additionally, he was the Rector of Imperial College from 2008 to 2009. Prior to his post at Imperial, Sir Roy was head of the Department of Zoology at the University of Oxford and served as Director of the Wellcome Trust Centre for the Epidemiology of Infectious Disease. His principal research interests are epidemiology, biomathematics, demography, parasitology, immunology, and health economics. His current research includes work on diseases, such as bovine spongiform encephalopathy in cattle, scrapie in sheep, and bovine tuberculosis in cattle. Sir Roy has also worked for the European Commission, the Canadian and U.S. governments, and the U.S. National Academies. He currently chairs the science advisory board of the World Health Organization's (WHO) Neglected Tropical Diseases (NTD) program, is a member of the Bill & Melinda Gates Foundation's Grand Challenges advisory board, and chairs the Schistosomiasis Control Initiative advisory board (SCI) funded by the Gates Foundation. Additionally, he is a non-executive director of GlaxoSmithKline. Sir Roy is a Founding Fellow of the Academy of Medical Sciences, a Foreign Associate Member of the U.S. Institute of Medicine, a Fellow of the Royal Society, a Foreign Member of the French Academy of Sciences, and was knighted in 2006.

Dr. Ilaria Capua, D.V.M., Ph.D.

Dr. Ilaria Capua is Director of the Research Department of Comparative Biomedical Sciences at the Istituto Zooprofilattico Sperimentale delle Venezie, Legnaro, Italy, which hosts the National, Food and Agriculture Organization (FAO), and World Organisation for Animal Health (OIE) Reference Laboratory for avian influenza and Newcastle disease, and the OIE Collaborating Centre for Diseases at the Human-Animal Interface. Her group of more than 70 staff provides diagnostic expertise globally and conducts cutting-edge research on influenza viruses and viral zoonoses. From 2005 to 2009, she was Chairman of OFFLU, the OIE/FAO network on animal influenza. In 2006, she launched the Global Initiative on Sharing All Influenza Data (GISAID) to share influenza virus sequences globally. Dr. Capua also has extensive experience coordinating international research projects funded by the European Commission (EC) and has worked closely with FAO managing

Technical Cooperation Projects covering 40 countries. She is a member of the World Health Organization's (WHO) Scientific and Technical Advisory Group on Influenza and a Stream leader within WHO's Global Research Agenda on Influenza. In 2007, she was among the winners of the Scientific American 50 prize; in 2008, she was included among Seed Magazine's Revolutionary Minds, for leadership in science policy; and she was the 2011 awardee of the Penn Vet World Leadership Award.

Dr. Michael Doyle, Ph.D.

Dr. Michael Doyle is Regents Professor of Food Microbiology and Director of the Center for Food Safety at the University of Georgia. His research focuses on bacterial foodborne pathogens including Escherichia coli O157:H7 and other serotypes of enterohemorrhagic E. coli, Salmonella spp., Campylobacter jejuni, Listeria monocytogenes, Staphylococcus aureus, and Clostridium botulinum. Dr. Doyle has more than 30 years of experience in Food Safety Research and Initiatives, and has published more than 400 scientific papers on food microbiology and food safety topics. Dr. Doyle holds the patents to several sanitation products developed at the University of Georgia. He was the recipient of a 2010 University of Georgia Research Foundation Inventor's Award for his invention of a food wash that significantly reduces the risk of foodborne illnesses. Additionally, in 1996, he received a Nicholas Appert Award of the Institute of Food Technologists (IFT) for preeminence in, and contributions to, the field of food technology. Dr. Doyle is a member of the Institute of Medicine of the National Academies and is the chair of the Institute of Medicine's Food Forum. He is a fellow of the American Academy of Microbiology, the International Association for Food Protection, and the IFT.

Dr. Robert Gallo, M.D.

Prof. Robert Gallo is Founder and Director of the Institute of Human Virology (IHV) at the University of Maryland. Prior to this role, he spent 30 years at the National Institutes of Health's National Cancer Institute, where he was head of its Laboratory of Tumor Cell Biology. Dr. Gallo is renowned for his research on HIV, most notably his co-discovery in 1984 that HIV is the cause of AIDS. His research has been instrumental in the development of HIV blood tests and HIV therapies. In 1996, his discovery that a natural compound known as chemokines can block HIV and halt the progression of AIDS was hailed by Science magazine as one of that year's most important scientific breakthroughs. Dr. Gallo's current work at the IHV combines the disciplines of research, patient care, and prevention programs in a concerted effort to speed the pace of medical breakthroughs. Dr. Gallo has authored more than 1,200 scientific publications, as well as the book "Virus Hunting: AIDS, Cancer & the Human Retrovirus: A Story of Scientific Discovery." Dr. Gallo has been awarded 29 honorary doctorates and was twice a recipient of the Albert Lasker Clinical Medical Research Award (1982 and 1986). He is a member of the National Academy of Sciences and the Institute of Medicine.

Dr. John Glass, Ph.D.
Dr. John Glass is a Professor in the Synthetic Biology Group at the J. Craig Venter Institute (JCVI), where he directs the Mycoplasma Biology team. He is also an adjunct faculty member of the University of Maryland at College Park Cellular and Molecular Biology Program. Prior to this role, he spent five years in the Infectious Diseases Research Division of the pharmaceutical company Eli Lilly, where he directed a Hepatitis C virology group and a microbial genomics group. At JCVI, Dr. Glass has led research on mycoplasma minimal genome and genome transplantation projects, as well as environmental genomics and viral metagenomics work. Notably, his team has been responsible for the creation of a synthetic bacterial cell. These developments are now being used to create cells and organelles with redesigned genomes to make microbes that can produce biofuels, pharmaceuticals, and industrially valuable molecules. In addition, Dr. Glass is currently leading a Venter Institute effort that uses synthetic genomics methods to improve the speed of production and efficacy of influenza virus vaccines.

Prof. Shaun Kennedy, B.S.Ch.E.
Prof. Shaun Kennedy is Director of the National Center for Food Protection and Defense (NCFPD). Additionally, he is the Director of Partnerships and External Relations of the University of Minnesota's College of Veterinary Medicine, and an Assistant Professor in the Department of Veterinary Population Medicine. Since joining the university, he has taken a leadership role in advancing research in animal health, food safety, and food-system biosecurity. Prior to these roles, Prof. Kennedy was the Vice President of Global Food and Beverage Research and Development at Ecolab, where he led his organization in developing a wide range of animal-health and food-safety technologies. These included novel sanitizers, FDA-approved process additives, new sanitation technologies, and animal health products. He has also held executive positions at Procter & Gamble. Prof. Kennedy provided the inaugural lecture in the Food and Drug Administration's (FDA) Chief Scientist Lecture series and has served on several European Commission projects on food-

system protection. Additionally, he received the FDA Commissioner's Special Citation for advancing food defense.

Prof. Joyce Tait, C.B.E., F.R.S.E., Ph.D.

Prof. Joyce Tait is the Innogen Scientific Advisor in the ESRC Innogen Centre, School of Social and Political Sciences at the University of Edinburgh. Previously, she was the Director of the Innogen Centre. Prof. Tait has an interdisciplinary background in natural and social sciences with concentrations in: developments in life sciences; strategic and operational decision-making in companies and public bodies; policy analysis; risk assessment and regulation; foresight; and public attitudes and communication. Her current research foci include genetically modified (GM) crops, cell therapies, the agro-biotechnology and pharmaceutical industries and their governance, and synthetic genomics. Prof. Tait is on the board of directors of the Scottish Stem Cell Network, a member of the board of the Roslin Foundation, and a member of the Scientific and Technical Council of the International Risk Governance Council. She has previously held appointments on a number of different bodies including the Nuffield Council on Bioethics, the Scottish Science Advisory Council, and the U.K. Food Standards Agency's GM Dialogue Steering Group. She is a fellow of the Royal Society of Edinburgh, a fellow of the Society for Risk Analysis, and has received a Commander of the British Empire (C.B.E.) award for her services to social science.

Prof. Kasisomayajula "Vish" Viswanath, Ph.D.

Prof. Vish Viswanath is an Associate Professor in the Department of Society, Human Development, and Health at the Harvard School of Public Health (HSPH) and in the Division of Population Sciences at the Dana-Farber Cancer Institute (DFCI). He is the Faculty Director of the Health Communication Core of the Dana-Farber/ Harvard Cancer Center (DF/HCC), and Co-Leader of the Cancer Risk and Disparities (CaRD) Program of DF/HCC. Prof. Viswanath also chairs the Steering Committee for the Health Communication Concentration at HSPH. His additional appointments include: Director, Enhancing Communication for Health Outcomes (ECHO) Laboratory, DF/HCC; and Associate Director, Lung Cancer Disparities Center, HSPH. His primary research is in documenting the relationship among communication inequalities, poverty, and health disparities. He has written more than 110 journal articles and book chapters concerning communication inequalities and health disparities, public health communication campaigns, e-health and the digital divide, public health preparedness, and the delivery of health communication interventions to underserved populations. He is the co-editor of three books: "Mass Media, Social Control and Social Change"; "Health Behavior and Health Education: Theory, Research, and Practice", and "The Role of Media in Promoting and Reducing Tobacco Use". Prof. Viswanath also is editor of the Communication and Social and Behavioral Change section of the 12-volume International Encyclopedia of Communication.

Biographical Information of ISGP Staff

George Atkinson, Ph.D.

Dr. George Atkinson is the founder and the Executive Director of the ISGP and remains Professor of Chemistry, Biochemistry, and Optical Science at the University of Arizona. His professional career spans several diverse arenas: academic teaching, research and administration, corporate founder and executive, and public service at the federal level. He is former head of the Department of Chemistry at the University of Arizona, the founder of a high-technology laser sensor company serving the semiconductor industry, and Science and Technology Adviser (STAS) to U.S. Secretaries of State Colin Powell and Condoleezza Rice. Notably, Dr. Atkinson also launched the Institute on Science for Global Policy (ISGP) in January 2008. The concepts and principles used by Dr. Atkinson to develop the ISGP derived from his personal experiences in domestic and international science policy. He seeks to guide the ISGP in creating a new type of international forum in which credible global experts provide governmental and societal leaders with the objective understanding of the science and technology (existing, emerging, and "at-the-horizon") now critically needed to formulate sound policy decisions. These are the Science and Technology (S&T) issues that can be reasonably anticipated to shape the increasingly global societies of the 21st century. His academic and professional achievements have been recognized in numerous ways including a National Academy of Sciences (NAS) Post Doctoral Fellowship at the National Bureau of Standards, Senior Fulbright Fellowship, an SERC Award (U.K.), the Senior Alexander von Humboldt Award (Germany), a Lady Davis Professorship (Israel), the first American Institute of Physics' Scientist Diplomat Award, the Distinguished Service Award (Indiana University), an Honorary Doctorate (Eckerd College), the Distinguished Achievement Award (University of California, Irvine), and selection by students as the Outstanding Teacher at the University of Arizona. He received his B.S. (high honors, Phi Beta Kappa) from Eckerd College and his Ph.D. in physical chemistry from Indiana University.

Jennifer Boice, M.B.A.

Jennifer Boice is the Program Manager of the ISGP. Prior to this role, Ms. Boice worked for 25 years in the newspaper industry, primarily at the Tucson Citizen and briefly at USAToday. She was the Editor of the Tucson Citizen when it was closed in 2009. Additional appointments at the Tucson Citizen included Business News Editor, Online Department head and Senior Editor. She also was a columnist.

Ms. Boice received an M.B.A. from the University of Arizona and graduated from Pomona College in California with a degree in economics.

Melanie Brickman Stynes, Ph.D., M.Sc.

Melanie Brickman Stynes is Associate Director for the Emerging and Persistent Infectious Diseases (EPID) program with the ISGP. As a researcher focused on the juncture of public health, demography, policy, and geography, she bridges multiple fields in her emerging and persistent infectious diseases research. Her work has paid particular attention to issues surrounding tuberculosis control (historic and contemporary). She is also an Adjunct Professor at Baruch College's School of Public Affairs in New York City. Additionally, Dr. Brickman Stynes spent nearly a decade as a Research Associate for the Center for International Earth Science Information Network (CIESIN) of Columbia University, where she worked on a range of projects related to health, disease, poverty, urbanization, and population issues. She received her Ph.D. in medical geography from University College London and her M.Sc. in medical demography from the London School of Hygiene and Tropical Medicine.

Jill Fromewick, Sc.D., M.S.

Jill Fromewick is Senior Scientific Consultant with the ISGP. A social epidemiologist by training, Dr. Fromewick maintains a dual focus on quantitative and qualitative methods. Her research spans a broad range of public health topics, primarily focused on investigating the impact of state and local policy on health and health disparities. She is the founder and Executive Director of Sparrow Research Group, a global public health consulting firm specializing in program design, evaluation, and social science research. Dr. Fromewick holds Master's and Doctor of Science degrees from the Department of Society, Human Development, and Health at the Harvard School of Public Health.

Jung Joo "JJ" Hwang, Ph.D., M.S., Pharm.D.

JJ Hwang is a Fellow with the ISGP. Dr. Hwang is a Consultant to the BioAtla, LLC and currently enrolled in a master's program at the University of California San Diego International Relations/Pacific Study, specializing in international public policy with a focus on global health. She has been a Scientific Director and Lab Head at Samsung Advanced Institute of Technology, a Scientific Director at Protedyne Inc., a Senior Scientist at MitoKor, and an Assistant Professor of Biochemistry and Molecular Biology at the University of Southern California, while managing various projects on biomarker/drug/diagnostic chip development. She received her Ph.D. in Biochemistry at the University of Pittsburgh School of Medicine and her M.S. and Pharm.D. from the Ewha Womans University in South Korea.

Anna Isaacs, M.Sc.

Anna Isaacs is Scientific/Program Consultant with the ISGP. She has previously focused on minority health issues and is experienced in primary and secondary qualitative research. Anna has interned as a researcher at a variety of nonprofit institutions and also at the House of Commons in London. She received her M.Sc. with distinction in Medical Anthropology from University College London and a B.Sc. in Political Science from the University of Bristol.

Brendan Lee, D.V.M, M.Sc., M.P.H., D.A.C.V.P.M.

Brendan Lee is Senior Scientific Consultant with the ISGP and a Research Fellow with the National Center for Food Protection and Defense at the University of Minnesota. After practicing clinical veterinary medicine for several years, he turned his focus to public health and food safety. Currently, his primary focus is on issues surrounding food safety, global food systems, and zoonotic diseases, with an emphasis on developing countries. He received his D.V.M. from the University of The West Indies, his M.Sc. in Veterinary Epidemiology and Public Health from the University of London, and his M.P.H. from the University of Minnesota.

David Miller, M.B.A.

David Miller is a Senior Fellow with the ISGP. Previously, he was Director, Medical Advocacy, Policy and Patient Programs at GlaxoSmithKline, where he led the company's U.S. efforts relating to science policy. In this role, he advised senior management on policy issues, and was the primary liaison between the company and the national trade associations, Pharmaceutical Research and Manufacturers of America (PhRMA) and Biotechnology Industry Organization (BIO). He also held management positions in business development and quality assurance operations. Mr. Miller received his B.S. in Chemistry and his M.B.A. from the University of North Carolina at Chapel Hill.

Arthur Rotstein, M.S.J.

Arthur Rotstein is the Media Coordinator for the ISGP. Prior to joining the ISGP, Mr. Rotstein worked for the Washington D.C. Daily News, held a fellowship at the

University of Chicago, and spent more than 35 years working as a journalist with The Associated Press. His writings have covered diverse topics that include politics, immigration, border issues, heart transplant and artificial heart developments, Biosphere 2, college athletics, features, papal visits, and the Mexico City earthquake. Mr. Rotstein holds a M.S.J. from Northwestern University's Medill School of Journalism.

Raymond Schmidt, Ph.D.

Ray Schmidt is a Senior Fellow with the ISGP. In addition, he is a physical chemist/ chemical engineer with a strong interest in organizational effectiveness and community health care outcomes. While teaching at the university level, his research focused on using laser light scattering to study liquids, polymer flow, and biological transport phenomena. Upon moving to the upstream petroleum industry, he concentrated on research and development (R&D) and leading multidisciplinary teams from numerous companies to investigate future enhanced oil recovery ideas and to pilot/commercialize innovative recovery methods in domestic and foreign locations. Dr. Schmidt received his Ph.D. in chemistry from Emory University.

Matt Wenham, D.Phil.

Matt Wenham is a Senior Fellow with the ISGP and a postdoctoral research fellow at the National Institutes of Health in Bethesda, Maryland. His research involves studying the interaction of protein toxins produced by pathogenic E. coli strains with human cells. Dr. Wenham received his D. Phil. from the Sir William Dunn School of Pathology, University of Oxford, United Kingdom, where he was a Rhodes Scholar. Prior to this, he worked in research positions at universities in Adelaide and Melbourne, Australia. Dr. Wenham received his bachelor's and honours degrees in biochemistry from the University of Adelaide, South Australia, and holds a Graduate Diploma of Education from Monash University, Victoria.